CW01498333

"Gigi Engle is one of the most trusted
a sexy, smart, and shame-free guide th
with confidence. Compassionate, acc
perfect guide into the world of kink. \
does it better than Gigi. This book em
and without shame. Whether you're dipping a toe or diving right in, Engle shows
that curiosity is not only welcome—it's essential."

—*Rachel Thompson, author of* Rough *and* The Love Fix

"*Kink Curious* isn't just accessible, it offers a step-by-step approach to removing
sexual shame and exploring all sorts of kinks, from mild to wild to fantastical. Let
Engle open your eyes (mouth, and holes) to a world of sexual possibilities."

—*Zachary Zane, author of* Boyslut: A Memoir and Manifesto

"*Kink Curious* is packed with the useful information that all kinksters need to know.
Gigi's warm and fun style centers on sex-positivity, dispelling common myths and
helping readers embrace their kink without shame. It is a must-read for all kinksters
whether curious, beginners, or more experienced."

—*Silva Neves, author of* Sexology: The Basics

"Nobody does it like Gigi Engle. In *Kink Curious*, she educates, delights, and validates
with characteristic moxy and deep intelligence. Her compassion for everyone and
anyone struggling with sexual shame shines in every paragraph. Read this book to
understand yourself and your species better."

—*Wednesday Martin, Ph.D., #1 New York Times bestselling author of*
Primates of Park Avenue *and* UNTRUE

"With humour and compassion, Engle makes the complex world of kink feel both
safe and exciting. This conversational guide has created an accessible entry to the
world of exploration that will serve curious beginners and seasoned players alike."

—*Dr. Esmé Louise James, historian and author of* Kinky History

"Gigi Engle is an expert I trust 100 percent to look after all kink-curious humans, from
their hearts to their intimate parts, their brains to their bruised bottoms and beyond!
This book snaps on a pair of elbow-length latex gloves and delves deep, intelligently
yet accessibly examining topics such as whether fetish practices can be used as a
form of therapy, how neurodiversity might intersect with kinky hobbies, and how
to enjoy imaginative role play without feeling like a fool or a fraud. If the thought
of something supposedly taboo secretly makes you think "Oooh...", and you want
a whip-smart, welcoming guide to kink that suits beginners but still goes beyond
the basics, *Kink Curious* will polish your knowledge to a glossy, rubberised shine."

—*Alix Fox, award-winning sex writer, journalist and broadcaster: The Guardian,*
*BBC Radio 1. Script Consultant for Netflix's* Sex Education

of related interest

**TRANS SEX**
A Guide for Adults
*Kelvin Sparks*
ISBN 978 1 83997 043 6
eISBN 978 1 83997 044 3

**QUEER SEX**
A Trans and Non-Binary Guide to
Intimacy, Pleasure and Relationships
*Juno Roche*
ISBN 978 1 78592 406 4
eISBN 978 1 78450 770 1

**HOW TO UNDERSTAND YOUR SEXUALITY**
A Practical Guide for Exploring Who You Are
*Meg-John Barker and Alex Iantaffi*
*Illustrated by Jules Scheele*
*Foreword by Erika Moen*
ISBN 978 1 78775 618 2
eISBN 978 1 78775 619 9

# KINK CURIOUS

## A Guide to Exploring Your Kinks, Dispelling Shame, and Staying Safe

### GIGI ENGLE

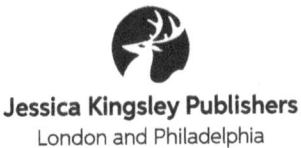

**Jessica Kingsley Publishers**
London and Philadelphia

First published in Great Britain in 2026 by Jessica Kingsley Publishers
An imprint of John Murray Press

1

Copyright © Gigi Engle 2026

Part of Chapter 1 was originally published as an article titled "A Beginner's
Guide to BDSM" in October 2024 on www.cosmopolitan.com
Part of Chapter 1 was originally published as an article titled "A Guide to the DD/
lg Dynamic in BDSM" in November 2023 on www.cosmopolitan.com
Part of Chapter 2 was originally published as an article titled "What is a
'Brat' in BDSM?" in February 2025 on www.menshealth.com
Part of Chapter 2 was originally published as an article titled "Here's What it Means
to Be Top, Vers, or Bottom" in July 2023 on www.cosmopolitan.com
Select parts of Chapter 4 were originally published as sections of articles titled "A Beginner's
Guide to Breeding Kink" and "How to do to Sensory Play" on www.cosmopolitan.com
Part of Chapter 6 was originally published as an article titled "What is Shibari? Here's
Everything You Need to Know" in October 2024 on www.cosmopolitan.com
Part of Chapter 7 was originally published as an article titled "How to Use Choking
During Sex, According to Experts" in June 2020 on www.menshealth.com
Part of Chapter 8 was originally published as an article titled "How Kink Can
Be Used to Help Your Mental Health" in February 2021 on www.TheBody.com
Part of Chapter 9 was originally published as an article titled "Exploring Your Erotic
Mind Can Improve Your Sex Life" in June 2022 on www.TheBody.com
Part of Chapter 13 was originally published as an article titled "The Importance
of Sexual Aftercare" in November 2022 on www.TheBody.com

Front cover image source: Kara McHale. The cover image is for illustrative
purposes only, and any person featuring is a model.

A CIP catalogue record for this title is available from the British Library and the Library of Congress

ISBN 978 1 80501 862 9
eISBN 978 1 80501 863 6

Printed and bound in Great Britain by Clays Ltd

Jessica Kingsley Publishers' policy is to use papers that are natural, renewable and recyclable
products and made from wood grown in sustainable forests. The logging and manufacturing
processes are expected to conform to the environmental regulations of the country of origin.

Jessica Kingsley Publishers
Carmelite House
50 Victoria Embankment
London EC4Y 0DZ

www.jkp.com

John Murray Press
Part of Hodder & Stoughton Ltd
An Hachette Company

The authorised representative in the EEA is Hachette Ireland,
8 Castlecourt Centre, Dublin 15, D15 XTP3, Ireland (email: info@hbgi.ie)

To everyone who has had taboo desires and wanted to venture down the path of sexual exploration.

And for Stepan, as always.

# ACKNOWLEDGMENTS

Writing this book has been a dream beyond my wildest imagination, and it is an honor and a privilege to have been able to share it with everyone.

Taking on this project was no easy feat, and I wouldn't have been able to do it without the love and support of the people I love and care about most. Thank you to my total dreamboat of a husband, Stepan, who proofread my entire manuscript more than once in order to make this book what it is. Thank you to my family, especially my sister and best friend, Chloe, who is always my biggest fan. Thank you to my best friends, Juli and Mary, for always being in my corner throughout this journey.

Thank you endlessly to all the brilliant and amazing experts in this book who so generously shared their knowledge with me. Without your insights, this book would not be what it is. I owe you all big time.

Thank you to my wonderful agent, Kara, for getting this book project on its path, and to my editor, Jane, for helping bring it to life. Thank you to JKP for helping turn this into a reality. It's been dreamy working with you.

And, finally, thank you to all you kink curious folx out there who are just beginning your journey. I hope you find something special and meaningful in these pages. You're the reason we're here.

I love you all and thank you for being on this adventure with me. Xoxo

# CONTENTS

*Introduction*                                                                 **9**

*Glossary*                                                                    **17**

## PART I. UNDERSTANDING KINK

1.  Intro to Kink                                                             **31**

2.  Powerplay: The Foundational Layer of Kink Play                           **45**

3.  Kink vs. Fetish                                                          **73**

4.  Understanding Kink: The Psychology of Play                              **87**

5.  The Intersections of Kink, Queerness, Gender Diversity,
    and Neurodiversity                                                      **107**

## PART II. KINK AND SEXUAL HEALTH

6.  Physical Safety: The Basics                                             **121**

7.  Emotional Safety: The Basics                                           **143**

8.  Kink as Therapy: How Some Folx Use Kink for Healing                    **177**

# PART III. INTEGRATION: EXPLORING YOUR AUTHENTIC KINKY SELF

9. Getting to the Bottom of Your Kinks and Tapping into the Erotic Mind      **189**

10. Dom? sub? Top? bottom? Switch? How To Embrace Your Authentic Kink Identity      **213**

11. Am I Broken?: How to Embrace Your Kinks and Fetishes in an Authentic Way      **251**

12. The Safety Container: Consent, Safe Words, Limits, Boundaries      **273**

13. Your Guide to Aftercare      **295**

14. Bringing a Partner into Your Kink Journey      **313**

*Further Reading and Resources*      **328**

*Bibliography*      **331**

# INTRODUCTION

Kink has been around since humans have existed. We're a kinky species, folx. We're curious and we love pleasure. Kink is deeply human at its core.

The ancient Greeks were well-known kinky freaks. As historian Dr. Esmé Louise James points out in her book *Kinky History*, this is highly documented. They absolutely loved dildos, strapons, pleasure, foot fetishes, and all things kinky. Did you know the oldest dildo is 28,000 years old? It was found in fragmented pieces in a cave in Germany. Its use is somewhat debated because the artifact predates the written word, but it's pretty damn clear that people were using this stone dildo to get their rocks off. Pun intended. I mean, it was "highly polished at the top from overuse" (James, 2024). Like, get real. Take me back, I say.

As James also notes, the Victorians were known for their love of spanking and choking, to the point where informational pamphlets had to be distributed to tell people to stop choking everyone left and right because people were getting hurt. All this spanking and choking business was known as "The English Vice." And while this term wasn't intended to be a good thing, I kind of love it.

In the 1800s–1900s, we started seeing kinks and fetishes being labeled and categorized—but don't get it twisted. When we started using actual terms around kinks and fetishes, it was for diagnostic purposes. Kink wasn't categorized to make people feel seen or to help people find community. It was not about empowerment or promoting joy. No, it was, as James points out, about diagnosing "perversion" and pathologizing human sexual behavior that didn't fall within the "normal" realm.

Throughout history, we've repeatedly seen humans embrace pleasure and kink and then forget it, deprioritize it, and/or shame it, only to "discover" it once again. We didn't just emerge freaky in the modern era. We've always been kinky. We've always been sexually adventurous. We've always been interested in pushing the boundaries of sexual expression. What's happening now is that we're finally giving kink its time in the sun. And we love having it out here, ready to be lifted into the light once again.

In today's social landscape, kink is often painted as something incredibly inaccessible and quite scary for the average person. It comes with a truly astonishing amount of misconceptions, myths, and problematic stereotypes in the media (looking at you, Christian Grey!). But these myths and misconceptions couldn't be further from the truth. Kink is available to everyone. With so many people suddenly finding themselves kink-curious, there has never been a better time for a mental health-focused guide to kink and BDSM.

Welcome to *Kink Curious*.

*Kink Curious* is a sex-positive, accessible, non-judgmental guide to kink. It is the map we all need today, leaving behind the classic kink guides of the early noughties to arm readers with a modern and more inclusive take on kink and safety. This straightforward guide is for curious beginners but can also serve as a foundational source for seasoned kink lovers who are continuing to expand their knowledge. The book outlines the basics of kink, with a special emphasis on myth-busting, safety (both emotional and physical), and dispelling shame.

It's time to pull back the curtain of mystery to create a welcoming space for anyone interested in exploring their kinky side. Kink is for everyone.

And who the hell am I to be writing this book? I'm Gigi Engle, also known as Auntie Gigi. I'm an investigative journalist with over a decade of experience in the sexual health and wellness space. I've been researching, writing, and practicing kink for most of my adult life. I'm also a certified sex and relationships psychotherapist with a special focus on gender, sexuality, and relationship diversity (GSRD).

Throughout my career, I have written and researched hundreds of articles on kink, fetish, and BDSM. In many ways, this book is a culmination of my years of experience in the sexual wellness field. It is a curated collection of the wisdom I have accumulated. None of this knowledge would be possible without the help of some of the world's most celebrated kink experts, mental health professionals, and leaders in sexual wellness. Through years and years and countless hours of interviews, these experts have generously lent me their expertise to enhance my work, and many of their voices are interwoven into this book.

And I'm just so excited to have it all here in one place. Every single kink question you've ever had will be answered right here, right now, in a judgment-free, straightforward way.

I started writing about sex in the mid-aughts, with a truly horrendous blog that was a massive TMI about my dating life. I do not know why people kept agreeing to date me when I was oversharing (badly written) accounts of my (mostly) orgasm-less sex life with the mediocre men I went out with. I actually cannot overstate what a horror show this blog truly was.

I got a job right out of college at a millennial website, where I quickly picked up any and all content centered on sexuality. To this day, my favorite line from that time comes from an article I wrote about trying to change the taste of your vagina (you cannot, by the way): I guess my dreams of a champagne-flavored pussy are over. I am nothing if not incredibly classy.

When I went freelance, I continued down the path of writing sexuality content. My lack of a filter and willingness to cover all the stuff deemed "seedy and weird" basically guaranteed a steady flow of assignments.

One day, one of my editors suggested that I write a piece on anal sex for *Teen Vogue*. Honestly, I didn't think twice about it. A scientific, research-backed anal sex explainer for a teen magazine. Sure. Why not? Teens deserve information that can keep them safe and informed. And I know people hate hearing this, but teens are having anal. Sorry, it's true.

People were not happy about the article. OK, that's an understatement. People lost their goddamn minds. At one point, I was called a sodomite on a Republican news channel. I wasn't aware we, in the year of our Lord 2017, were still using the word "sodomite," but there it was on national television. A popular YouTuber and known neo-Nazi also hosted a book burning of *Teen Vogue*'s print edition. And yes, this was extreme, but I just can't believe she thought I was in print. It was truly a beautiful moment, honestly.

I got massively trolled. At times it was scary, and at times it was really funny. The joke was on the trolls because after I got a book deal, I wrote a whole guide about sex and embracing your gorgeous, slutty self.

What I learned from this absolute shit show was that people are seriously lacking in sex education. People are scared to death of good sexual health information. I learned that people in power were going to do everything they could to keep good, empowering information away from the general public. And it solidified my purpose: I needed to fight even harder to provide good, science-backed sexual health information. I became certified in sex education, and I kept right on rolling.

It was while writing my first book, *All The F\*cking Mistakes:*

*A Guide to Sex, Love, and Life*, that I realized that I was, in fact, incredibly queer. I, a person who had been writing about sex on the internet for over five years at that point, a person who proudly wrote about the power of sexual freedom and tearing down the patriarchy, was harboring an immense amount of internalized biphobia. On top of this, I figured out I was also very, very kinky. What a revelation. I was a *very, very* bisexual, kinky woman with a passion for bisexual chaos and all things a wee bit freaky.

Embracing who I truly am was a pivotal moment in my personal and professional development. It armed me with a new community and a whole new world of sexual freedom to explore. It was pretty magical.

At 30, I decided to pursue training in sex therapy with a focus on the gender, sexuality, and relationship-diverse population so that other little queers like me wouldn't spend the first 27 years of their lives wondering if they had any right to be queer at all. I wanted to help other confused queer girls, boys, and people to feel comfortable in their skin. I wanted to take on all the kinksters and the non-monogamous babes and let them know they were valid and amazing. I wanted to create a space for truly sex-positive therapy where people could come and open up without shame in a way that felt authentic. Sexuality is a tender subject. It deserves to be handled gently.

So, because of this wild, sexy, weird journey to where I am today, I decided to create a trauma-informed, sex-positive, mental health-focused kink guidebook for the gorgeous, anxious over-thinkers among us. Because with so much "fifty-shades-esque" garbage crowding the internet, the media constantly equating BDSM with abuse and harm, and the regular pathologizing of folx who have diverse sexual interests, there are few places for the curious kinkster to turn. We all deserve better.

Before we begin discussing sex and kink, I have to acknowledge my privilege as a white, middle-class, straight-presenting, gender-flexible femme. I will not get everything right for every single person, and some of what I say may not gel with every person's belief system. I want to hold myself accountable as a professional in this space who is still very fallible. I'm going to do my very, very best to be inclusive, nuanced, and loving while we deep-dive into these sensitive (and sexy!) topics.

It's also very important to acknowledge that there are many intersections with kink and queerness, BIPOC (Black, Indigenous, and people of color) folx, neurodivergent, and gender-diverse populations. While there is a chapter dedicated to these intersections, this book aims to be inclusive throughout, including a wide variety of interviews with interdisciplinary kink experts across the globe. The goal is to allow the voices of marginalized folx to shine because they are largely why kink is the marvelous and self-actualizing practice that it is.

This book serves as a roadmap to guide you on your journey into the land of the sexual taboo and aims to help anyone and everyone feel more at home in their bodies and sexuality.

To fully embrace, accept, and enjoy kink, we have to lay a foundation of care around our emotional and physical health. While kink can be deeply pleasurable, healing, and a tool of self-discovery, it needs to be done within a context of education, negotiation, and mutual respect. This book will serve as a guide to take even the most anxious kink-curious folx to a place of solid understanding and comfort in their practice. Kink is not all about whips and chains and spanking—it is about exploring the human condition, power dynamics, and one's capacity for pleasure in the realm of the taboo.

The kink community has a long-held history of upholding

pillars of consent and safety within play. Vanilla folx—that is, those who don't indulge in kink—aren't taught these tenets as a part of being a sexually considerate person. The lessons in this book can be applied to any kind of sex to infuse it with consideration, empathy, and respect.

The book is broken down into three main sections. Each section is designed to equip you with the tools you need before moving on to the next phase of your kinky journey. Part I is a crash course in kink basics—because, frankly, we all need that in our lives. It is your 101 guide to understanding some of the key terms and concepts of kink. It serves as a foundational learning platform to equip you with the knowledge you need to practice kink in a safe way. We'll take a deep dive into what kink is (and what it isn't), we'll learn about the foundational dynamic in kink (powerplay), we'll explore different kinky roles and how these play out in real life, and take a look at how kink serves marginalized communities and acts as a means of self-actualization for many in the queer and gender-diverse populations.

Part II is where we get really hot and heavy with our mental and physical health. Kink is such a beautiful way to explore the vast expansiveness of our sexuality and identity, but it needs to be done with caution and care. We'll start with physical safety. You'll learn all the basics and how to hone your craft to have truly amazing kink experiences. Next, we'll venture into emotional and mental safety, consent, and how kink can be used therapeutically for those who love it. Kink isn't therapy, but that doesn't mean it isn't healing. This is a hill I will die on.

Part III is where we get juicy. It's time to learn how to use kink to explore your authentic, sexy self. Part III is where we, now fully loaded with newfound kink knowledge, can take what we've acquired and apply it to our own lives in a way that feels safe and healthy for us as individuals. We'll start with figuring out your kinks and tapping into the erotic mind, then move into embracing and discovering the kinky role (or roles!) that suits you best. You'll learn how to wrangle all we've learned about safe words, consent, aftercare, and more into a framework for your practice. And last, you'll learn how to invite a partner to explore kink with you.

Throughout the book, you'll find worksheets, journal prompts, and other exercises that are designed to enhance your learning. These aren't mandatory (we're all about consent here), but they can serve as tools to help you delve deep into your desires and wants so you can start to form a clearer understanding of how kink can be integrated into your life. I've found that homework and exercises have helped many of my clients discover and embrace their authentic kinky selves, and I'm hoping you'll benefit from this hands-on learning style, too. I'm very conscious that some curious kinksters may be neurodivergent or may prefer not to write things down. Feel free to customize exercises in any style that works for you, whether that be by recording voice notes, drawing, or creating broader thought collections.

You'll also find various "Agony Aunt" letters in which I harness my signature Auntie Gigi style to thoroughly answer some of the more common questions I've received from clients and readers alike. And let's be real, who doesn't love an advice letter?

This is going to be such a beautiful journey, and I promise that we are going to have So Much Fun.

# GLOSSARY

This book is not what anyone would ever deem "term light." There are a lot of words, phrases, terms, and concepts specific to kink that might leave you confused and ready to slam this guide shut and run out into a field to scream into the sky. That's just not what I want for you, my beauty.

This is why I have put together this handy-dandy glossary of terms. I don't want to interrupt your reading too much, so if you come across a word or phrase that doesn't make sense to you, simply flip back to this section and it will be explained concisely and straightforwardly. All terms are in alphabetical order for ease.

You may also choose to read through these terms before we plunge into the world of kink. It's totally up to you.

Let's do it.

### AMAB
AMAB stands for "assigned male at birth." This is an inclusive term used for people who were assigned male at birth, including cisgender men. A person's assigned sex at birth may not correspond with their gender identity. This term refers to how society perceives us at birth.

### AFAB
AFAB stands for "assigned female at birth." This is an inclusive term used for people who were assigned female at birth and cis-female folx. A person's assigned sex at birth may not correspond with

their gender identity. This term refers to how society perceives us at birth.

## AFTERCARE

Aftercare is the way we nurture and care for ourselves and our partners after sexual play finishes. Aftercare is a set of actions and activities consensually agreed upon before sex (or the scene) begins. It is a post-sex plan of action to ensure that everyone involved in the play feels safe and well taken care of. This can include cuddling, having a cup of tea, discussing the scene, brushing hair, and anything else that works for you.

## ALIEN IMPLANTATION FETISH

Alien implantation fetish is a type of role-play in which a person is "bred" by aliens. This is a subset of abduction fantasy. This can involve ovipositors, devices used to implant jelly eggs inside participants.

## ASEXUAL

Asexual refers to people who do not experience sexual attraction. Some asexual folx may experience some sexual attraction or desire, but only in certain contexts. Asexuality is a spectrum (known as the "ace spectrum"), and those who identify on the spectrum will vary widely in the way their asexuality manifests for them as individuals.

## BDSM

BDSM is an acronym that stands for bondage/discipline, Dominance/submission, and sadomasochism. BDSM encompasses a wide variety of practices involving intentional play with power dynamics and often intense sensations such as pain. BDSM can include role-play, fetish, and other practices that aren't considered "typical." "Typical" being heteronormative, vanilla sex.

## BOTTOM

Bottoming is a fun and interesting role to play during sex and erotic play. It has two meanings. 1. A bottom is the receiver during anal penetration, usually within the context of MLM sex. 2. A bottom is the receiver (or submissive) in kink play. The bottom is typically the person having things "done" to them.

## BOUNDARY

A boundary, also referred to as a "limit," refers to acts, words, etc. that are acceptable to a partner during kink play (and all forms of sex). The boundary denotes the parameters of play. Boundaries are used to create safe containers and to ensure everyone feels comfortable at all times during a scene.

## BRAT

A brat is a type of submissive in a D/s dynamic. A brat intentionally misbehaves to get a rise out of their Dom, often eliciting "punishments." The brat enjoys driving the Dom a bit mad with their naughtiness. It's all centered around defying authority, which can be very hot.

## BRAT TAMER

A Brat Tamer is the Dom in the brat/Brat Tamer dynamic. They may choose to go by a different name (like Sir, Daddy, Mommy, etc.), but the Brat Tamer is their *style* of Domination. Their role is to put the brat in their place, remind them of the rules, and enforce the punishments/orders that they have created together. It's an authoritative role.

## COCK AND BALL TORTURE (CBT)

Cock and ball torture refers to when a penis-owning submissive (usually a cisgendered man, but not always), enjoys having their cock and balls, well, tortured. It usually involves pain play and/or constriction of the penis/balls. This can happen in a variety of ways, including wearing chastity cages that prevent erections or having their balls stepped on in high heels.

## CNC

CNC stands for "consensual non-consent." CNC is a rape or ravishment fantasy. All parties involved are 100 percent consenting to the play.

## DENTAL DAM

A dental dam is a barrier method that goes inside the vagina. They are often called "female condoms." They are used to prevent pregnancy and the spread of STIs.

## DOM

The Dom or "Dominant" is the partner who is doing the "doing" during a kink scene. Doms usually engage in kink scenes that are BDSM-based, but not always. Being a Dom simply means you're the Top partner, the one who is consensually taking control from the submissive. Some women, femme, and AFAB folx may prefer the feminine version Domme, but everyone is different and will use the term that feels most authentic to them, regardless of sex or gender. In this book, I've chosen to use "Dom," as I've found that a lot of people use it, regardless of gender identity.

## DOMINATRIX

A professional Dom for whom being a Dom is their career. A Dominatrix usually refers to a cis-woman or femme.

### D/S DYNAMIC
The Dom/sub dynamic is most explicit when we're talking about kink and BDSM. This is when two or more people engage in consensual power exchange, usually in a BDSM context. The sub willingly hands over the power within the scene to the Dominant.

### ENTHUSIASTIC CONSENT
Enthusiastic consent means that you are giving a "hell yes" to a sexual or intimate act. You are giving your yes with excitement.

### ENTHUSIASTIC MAYBE
An enthusiastic maybe is when you give consent to try something you're not entirely sure if you're into quite yet. You're still open to trying said thing—excited, even—but you're leaving room for the nuance that comes when you're exploring something new. As with all forms of consent, it should be freely given and able to be revoked at any time, without physical or emotional consequences.

### EXHIBITIONISM
The sexual interest in being watched by others while engaging in sexual activity.

### FETISH
A fetish is something that doesn't "normally" constitute something typically "sexy." It is usually a non-sexual object or body part that a person finds sexually arousing. A fetish is when something that isn't normally equated with sexuality or sexual attraction brings a person sexual feelings. The types of fetishes that exist are extremely varied. Usually, when someone has a fetish, they require the fetish act or object to be present to achieve full sexual satisfaction.

**FURRY**
Furries are people who enjoy dressing up in elaborate animal costumes. Furries enjoy being animal characters in their role-play, often in conjunction with human characteristics. This can be a part of D/s play, but also a 24/7 lifestyle.

**GENDER BINARY**
The gender binary refers to the notion that people are classified on a binary of either male or female. Proponents of the gender binary believe there are only two genders and equate gender with biological sex. This is inaccurate, as sex is a component of biology, and gender is a social construct that exists on a spectrum.

**GENDER NON-CONFORMING, GENDER FLUID, GENDER FLUX, NON-BINARY (OR NB)**
These inclusive terms refer to folx who don't fall on the gender binary of "man/woman" that exist within our culture (and is a construct). The term(s) folx use and how they specifically define it will depend on what feels right for them.

**HUCOW**
HuCow stands for Human Cow fetish. This is a subset of breeding kink and animal role-play. The reasons people like HuCow are the transgressive themes, escapism, group sex, and body transformation. In this fetish, a person (or persons) plays a cow and is "bred" by a Dominant partner or group of people.

**IMPERIAL ORGY**
An orgy is a group sex experience. An imperial orgy refers to one that centers on a king/queen/empress/ruler who is the center of the

orgy—they are usually an object of sexual worship. An imperial orgy is one of many elaborate kink scenes that people can engage in.

### KINK

Kink is the catch-all umbrella term for all forms of non-vanilla intimate activity. Kink can involve a much wider range of activities, whereas BDSM focuses specifically on dynamics within bondage/discipline, Dominance/submission, and sadomasochism.

### MASOCHIST

A masochist is someone who enjoys and is aroused by intense pain being inflicted on them. This pain can be physical, psychological, or both.

### MLM

MLM stands for "men loving men." MLM usually refers to gay, pan, or bisexual men who are attracted to other men.

### NEURODIVERGENT

Neurodivergent means that your brain functions differently from a typical brain. This means you have different strengths and challenges from someone with a typical brain. Some examples of neurodivergence include ADHD, autism, OCD, and more.

### NEUROTYPICAL

Neurotypical means that your brain functions in a typical way. It usually refers to folx whose brains function in the way society expects.

### PEGGING

In its original form, pegging is when a person with a penis is anally penetrated by a person wearing a strap-on and dildo. The term has since become more inclusive to include any person who is anally penetrated by a person wearing a strap-on and/or dildo.

## PLAY
Play refers to all sexual and intimate acts and dynamics that take place between partners. Sex and kink are manifestations of how adults play with one another, hence the name. Play can include BDSM scenes, role-play, vanilla sex, and much more.

## POWER DYNAMICS
Power dynamics are the foundational layer of kink. They can look like the Dom/sub dynamic, a Top/bottom dynamic, and much more. In power dynamics, one partner consensually and enthusiastically gives power to the other(s).

## PRAISE KINK
When a person gets sexually aroused when someone gives them compliments, positive feedback, and/or sexual affirmations and praise. Getting a compliment and feeling great about that is one thing, but being legitimately turned the hell on is another. These kinks are all about using praise or positive reinforcement as a means of dominance in D/s dynamics.

## QUEER
Queer refers to sexual or gender identity that does not correspond to established ideas of sexuality and gender, specifically those that fall under heterosexual and cisgender norms. It has been considered a slur in the past but has been reclaimed by the queer community.

**RACK**

RACK stands for "risk awareness consensual kink." It is the framework for ethical kink practice. It ensures that everyone involved in a scene is aware of the risks of the play involved, consents to the play, and feels safe to engage authentically.

**SADIST**

A sadist is someone who derives sexual gratification from inflicting pain on others. In kink, this pain is inflicted consensually.

**SAFE GESTURES**

Safe gestures are non-verbal signals that mean a boundary or limit has been reached during a kink scene. These are usually employed when a partner's ability to speak is restricted, but not always. This will depend on the preferences of the people involved in the play—for example, three taps on your partner's body or some other surface.

**SAFE WORD**

A safe word is a word (or phrase) that is used to denote when a boundary or limit has been reached during a kink scene. It means you'd like the play to stop or pause. These words are usually non-sexual for clarity and safety. Some examples include red, sailboat, meatloaf (because I'd do anything for love, but I won't do that), windmill, etc. Safe words should be respected immediately by all partners.

**SCENE**

A scene is the context in which play happens. It is the container for partners to play in. A scene can look like role-play, BDSM, and much more. Put simply, a scene is the setting where an activity takes place, as well as the activity itself.

## SHIBARI
Shibari, or Kinbaku, is the art of Japanese rope tying. It is one of the "B's" in BDSM—bondage. Kinbaku means "tight binding," and Shibari means "tying."

## SPLOSHING
A fetish for jelly-like or messy substances. It is sometimes referred to as a "wet and messy fetish." Examples of sploshing include cake sitting, playing with Jell-O, and food play.

## SERVICE TOP
A service Top is someone who is a Top, but is in "service" to the other person's pleasure. They primarily enjoy doing sexual and kinky things to their partner based entirely on their pleasure. They enjoy the act of giving pleasure as a primary function of their own pleasure.

## SUB
The sub or "submissive" partner is the bottom in a D/s dynamic. A sub usually appears in a BDSM context, but not always. They are the partner who is having things done to them in a scene.

## SUB SPACE/DOM SPACE
sub space/Dom space refers to the meditative or transcendent experience that a sub or Dom may have during a kink scene. It is often equated to a "flow state," similar to those achieved in meditative practice or during intense exercise.

**TOP**

A Top is the person who is doing the "doing." This often means the giver of anal penetration within a MLM context, but it can also exist in all forms of sex. It's about power exchange. A Top may sometimes also be a Dom, but not always. Tops and bottoms both have a special place in queer and gender non-conforming sexual dynamics.

**VANILLA**

Vanilla refers to sex that falls within the "typical" range of sexual behaviors. These include penis-in-vagina sex, oral sex, etc. Vanilla refers to what society would deem as "normal" sex. Vanilla sex is sex that is not kinky.

**VERS**

Vers usually means you're interested in Topping and bottoming—and/or Domming and subbing. You're flexible in your kink role, usually depending on the context and acts involved. A person can be vers and have a strong preference for being a Top/bottom or Dom/sub.

**VOYEURISM**

The sexual interest in watching others engage in sexual activity.

**WLW**

This stands for "women loving women." It refers to women who are attracted to other women. This term is inclusive of lesbian, bisexual, and pansexual women, and non-binary people who identify with the social concept of womanhood.

## 24/7 DOM/SUB DYNAMIC

In a 24/7 dynamic, Doms and subs stay in their roles 100 percent of the time. Being in their Dom/sub dynamic is a part of their lifestyle rather than just a form of play in kink scenes.

# PART I

# UNDERSTANDING KINK

# 1

## INTRO TO KINK

**What you'll find in this chapter:**

→ What even is kink?

→ Why are people into it?

→ How people develop kinks.

→ A myth-busting section to dispel common worries: Does wanting to engage in kink mean you have a mental illness or trauma? Is all kink abuse?

→ Who is kink for? Can anyone get kink-alicious?

To know kink is to love kink—at least in my opinion. Kink is truly a term that is ever-evolving as it makes its mark on mainstream society. While they are quite an inaccurate portrayal of safe and consensual kink, the *Fifty Shades* books did a service to the BDSM and kink community that can't be denied. There are many other—far superior—media representations of kink, but none of them were able to bring BDSM out of the fringe and right to our front door in the same way Ana and Christian's story did. The books were a catalyst that allowed many people to *begin* to become kink curious. I doubt *this* book would exist if BDSM hadn't skyrocketed into the social narrative the way it has in the last ten years. So I do begrudgingly have to thank *Fifty Shades* for being a conversation starter and for offering us a place to begin a real, authentic journey into kink, one that embraces boundaries, consent, and personal freedom.

Perhaps kink should be written about by people who know and understand it in all its heady nuances. Shall we begin?

Kink is defined as "having unusual sexual interests." Meaning it is all sexual and sensual expression that falls outside of the socially prescribed, cisgender, heterosexual norm. When I say "cisgender, heterosexual norm," I mean any kind of sex that falls outside of penis-in-vagina intercourse. I mean any kind of sex that isn't about "making babies." You might be asking, "Wait, Gigi. If you're painting with such a broad brush, wouldn't things like oral sex, handjobs, and fingering be considered kinky?"

And the answer is "maybe." Usually, when we're talking about kink, we're not including acts like fingering, using a vibrator, oral sex, etc.—but this isn't strictly true for everyone, because what is kinky is in the eye of the beholder.

For one person, French kissing might be the kinkiest, wildest thing in the entire world. For another, being tied up, spat on, and called a dirty little slut might just be an average Tuesday evening. All of this is to say that kinkiness is more of a state of mind than a set of behaviors.

Since this is a guide to kink—one that aims to offer trauma-informed, hand-holding guidance—and I am your trusty navigator, we wouldn't be doing ourselves any favors by leaving kink in such an airy-fairy state. So let's rediscover kink.

After interviewing experts from across the broad kink spectrum—from professional BDSM practitioners to Shibari instructors, to curious devotees, to kinky sex workers, to psychologists, and mental health professionals who specialize in working with kinky clients—I aimed to capture what kink truly is. I was able to come up with the following loose definition. Kink is a form of self-expression that falls outside the social norm. As self-expression, it contains no bounds, while at the same time, it provides a safe container for you to explore your darkest desires, always knowing there are boundaries in place and a stop button with your safe word. Kink comes alive when you believe in it. Kink is a place to explore things that scare you in a way that invites agency and reclamation. Kink is transgressive. Kink is a journey.

I asked Dr. Lee Phillips, Ed.D., a psychotherapist and certified sex and couples therapist who works with kinky clients, how he would define kinky behaviors specifically. He agreed that trying to define kink is a challenging task. "Kink is best described as sexual behaviors and preferences that are not easily categorized or different from what we consider typical sexual interests. For example, a typical sexual interest, also known as 'vanilla sex,' would include kissing in a missionary position," he says. "Kinky sex may involve role-playing where one partner is submissive (the sub), and the other one is dominant (the Dom)."

Kink is best described as an "umbrella" term that covers a

rich and abundant group of sexual preferences. Kink is often
used interchangeably with BDSM by kinksters and the media
alike. While much of kink revolves around BDSM play, kink is
much more expansive than bondage, dominance, submission, and
sadomasochism. BDSM is kink, but kink isn't always BDSM. Kink
is a larger, more inclusive term under which BDSM falls.

Kinky sexual practices include, but are by no means limited
to, BDSM, fetishes, erotic role-play, and essentially any kind of
erotic behavior that might be called "transgressive" or "wrong"
by a fire-and-brimstone pastor standing at the front of a mega-
church—basically, everything that is pleasurable and naughty.
"Kink can be defined as sexual behaviors, sexual interests, or
relationship structures not accepted by the dominant culture,"
Phillips continues. "For example, a praise kink would be outside
of the norm regarding sexual activity because praise can involve
erotic role play (i.e., a little girl pleasing her daddy)."

What's more, when I asked kink educator Emerson Karsh how
she would define kink, she said it isn't just about sexual behaviors.
It can also include many forms of intimacy, relationship styles,
and sensual activities—all of which center on the consensual
power-exchange relationship. In power exchange, one partner
consensually hands power over to the other partner to create a
certain shared experience. It is a chance to play with giving and
receiving. As a submissive, you're allowing things to be done to you,
but you always know you're in control. There is a special intensity
in this dynamic because it allows us to fully express ourselves in a
safe way, free from the shackles of shame and judgment.

Not all kink is sexual, but all kink *is* intimate in some way.
That might just be the kicker, so let's say that again: Not all kink is
sexual, but all kink *is* intimate in some way. Kinkster Mistress Kye,
a professional Dominatrix, agrees, telling me in an interview that

"kink is purposeful intimacy that connects you with your shadow self in a truthful, vulnerable, brave and fulfilling way." Like, come on. That is beautiful.

Kink is:

- a journey
- a chance to be your true sexual self
- a place for exploration
- self-expression
- BDSM, role-play, sensory play, and other non-vanilla activities
- rooted in consensual power exchange
- rooted in boundaries, negotiation, and consent
- a normal part of human sexual expression.

Kink is not:

- all about whips and chains
- *Fifty Shades of Grey*
- inaccessible for people who don't have personal dungeons
- non-consensual
- expensive, if you don't want it to be (and it doesn't even need to include any gear)

+ only for weirdos or freaks

+ for people who like hurting others

+ only for people who have a lot of trauma

+ anything to be ashamed of.

## WHY ARE PEOPLE INTO KINK?

Why are people into kink, and why can't they just, like, be normal or whatever? Well, humans aren't normal. As I said in the intro to this book, we humans have been kinking it up since we figured out how to stand upright (and probably before that even). I'd invite anyone who says to themselves, "Oh, kink isn't for me. I'm a normal person who's fine having normal sex," to ask themselves why. Why is this a good thing? What is preferable or better about wanting to have vanilla sex over kinky experiences?

I asked Eva Oh, a professional Dominatrix, what unites people who enjoy kink. She told me that kink does not have to be related to trauma or psychological twists and turns, but what you will likely find is that a common theme for people who practice kink is an openness to experience.

Basically, we're into kink because we're freaky and curious.

Many people are into kink because of the taboo and transgressive themes that come with the play. We're turned on by the taboo. The more we're told by society not to want something, the more sexual and erotic power it takes on.

"It's important for non-kinksters to understand that the goal of everyone engaging in kink is pleasure," says Mistress Kye. "It's about exploring fantasies that make all parties feel good and oftentimes empowered. Sometimes, it's hard for non-kinksters to remember that everyone derives pleasure differently." And yeah, some people do derive pleasure from having their butt cheeks smacked to the high heavens with a paddle. Some people enjoy pain as a pathway to pleasure. Others might derive pleasure from filling up a bathtub with Jell-O and sitting in it while masturbating, or swimming around in it. (Note: If you do this, please use sugar-free Jell-O so you don't wind up with a raging yeast infection.)

People are into kink for one common reason: It's fun. It is as simple as that.

## WHERE DO KINKS COME FROM?

Pinpointing where a kink comes from is not an easy task. The reasons we find something sexually or sensually arousing are entirely subjective.

According to Karsh:

When thinking psychologically, people are into kink either due to intrinsic or extrinsic motivation. For some, it may stem from a lifelong interest, whereas for others, the interest in kink comes extrinsically. Some studies suggest that individuals who identify as kinksters or fetishists develop their interests during puberty, with some recognizing them as early as 13 years old, or even earlier in some cases. For those who are extrinsically motivated, kink becomes an interest later in life in response to outside motivations like positive experiences with a partner introducing it to you, a new form of expression or stress relief, arousal from positive or negative reinforcement, or to meet some newfound need or desire discovered through erotica.

You might discover that tickling is sexually arousing through experiences in childhood, or perhaps you discover this later in life during a tickle fight with a partner. You might find that vampire stories begin to form the basis for your fantasy life in puberty, or maybe you come to love blood and the undead in your 40s. Everyone is different.

When I asked Eva Oh about the psychological origins of kink, she agreed that it varies. She says that sometimes people can point to certain images and experiences that showed them they were into something, but not everyone has this. There aren't always pinpoint moments.

For Oh, kink is simply fun. It's an opportunity to be creative— spontaneously creative. It's more than just the tools and toys; it's about how one needs to consider how they should react and how they can react in any given scene. It's a bit like improv theater on an emotional level. It's an opportunity for Oh to experience her humanness in a more textured way. If you're comfortable with your fear and you want to experience it, that can be very good to understand about yourself. Kinks are a tool for self-exploration and deeper self-understanding.

She also wants people to know that it can just be a good time. Sure, it can be meaningful and beautiful, but it's just a very fun way to experience the world. Exploring kink can allow you to have a wider imagination over time. It has the potential to open up your human experience to things that you could be lacking if you're fearful or stay stuck in a place of shame.

No matter where a kink comes from or why you want to engage in it, we absolutely need to understand that it's all normal and healthy and fine and OK and neutral.

We only think that kink and "non-normative" sexual behaviors are bad and shameful because society tells us they're bad and shameful. Nothing about kink is inherently wrong or bad. It's all about social perception. Kink gets really bad PR. A lot of my work with clients is about unpacking and unraveling this deeply rooted shame around their kinks that comes from religious conservative messaging (though I'd argue most facets of society demonize kink). When we're able to untangle what is authentic for the client, rather than a message that was fed to them against their will, that is where true freedom and peace are found.

Once you realize you're not a bad person for enjoying spanking, bondage, or whatever else tickles your fancy, you are free. Even if kink is not your cup of tea, I'd argue that this continuous striving for sexual freedom is something we should all prioritize. Who has time for shame and stigma when there is so much pleasure and joy to be found in the world?

## WHO IS KINK FOR?

Kink is, ahem, for everyone. Seriously. Anyone can do this. Media representations of kink regularly make it feel like this inaccessible, scary, intimidating thing—but it doesn't have to be. All it takes to be kinky is a willingness to explore sexually in the realm of the taboo. If you're open to trying some "freaky" things in the bedroom, you're very much a candidate for the kink party. "Exploring kink provides people with an opportunity for self-reflection, challenge, and personal growth," Phillips says. "It provides a sacred space where people feel safe to try new things, push boundaries, flirt with edges, and conquer fears."

When we start to reframe kink as an opportunity for self-discovery rather than something only weirdos engage in, "The Red Room of Pain," we can finally start to give it the credit it deserves. "Kink can be whatever you want it to be," Karsh adds. "Kink can range from something as simple as receiving a birthday spanking to something as complex as engaging in 24/7 collared dynamics. It is a big, large, malleable, expressive range of anything you want."

It doesn't matter who you are, where you come from, how old you are, or anything else—kink is for *you*.

## FIVE MYTHS AND MISCONCEPTIONS ABOUT KINK

It's not a secret that we live in a pretty sex-negative culture. We constantly receive messages that sex is dirty and bad. Especially when it comes to sex that falls outside of the socially prescribed, very heteronormative framework, then phew, there is a lot of misinformation.

Let's unpack some of the misunderstandings that people have about BDSM because being armed with information can make play much more accessible—and less scary.

### 1. Only traumatized people want to engage in BDSM

There is nothing *wrong* with you if you want to try BDSM. You're just a person with a rich fantasy life. According to a 2008 study published in the *Journal of Sexual Medicine*, people who engage in BDSM are no more depraved or psychologically "damaged" than anyone else. "The notion that only traumatized people like BDSM is harmful, considering that BDSM is a very normal human behavior," kink expert Julieta Chiara told me in a recent interview.

### 2. Kink is abuse

God, this one is thrown around so much that it is *unreal*. This is "usually the perception of those who know very little or nothing about how things work in BDSM/kink. A million words cannot stop abuse. One word can stop a BDSM/kink scene. The difference is communication, negotiation, trust and explicit consent," Kye says.

BDSM is all about consent, boundaries, and positive intent. "Partners negotiate their boundaries and agree to what they are going to do before they do it," says Dr. Celina Criss, a sex coach specializing in kink. While accidents may happen (we're all humans capable of making mistakes), there is no intent to cause harm or injury to your partner.

"Responsible partners have safety protocols in place to prevent this from happening before, during, [and] after any scene," Criss continues. "This means they know what they're doing and the risks involved. They've practiced, learned about anatomy and physiology, keep their first-aid skills up to date, use safe words, and know what sort of aftercare their partner needs."

So, enough with the tired "BDSM is abuse" trope, because it is not accurate and, honestly, super harmful.

### 3. You must like pain to enjoy BDSM

"Almost all BDSM can be modified to be done without experiencing any pain at all," Chiara says. BDSM is about powerplay dynamics. While pain can be a part of it, it doesn't have to be. For example, you might enjoy being blindfolded and having a feather run all over your body by your Dom. It's not painful, but it's still BDSM.

What's more, Criss says that pain isn't a useful metric in BDSM and that most practitioners don't even measure sensation this way. "The experience of pain varies from person to person, and day to day," she explains. "It's more accurate to consider *intense sensation* to describe what is experienced by the partners. Intense sensation could be thuddy, stingy, or even feather-light."

## 4. BDSM is a fetish

BDSM are wider practices *within* a kink umbrella that express our needs and interests (sexual or non-sexual), while a fetish is an act or an item that we *must* have to be aroused/get to our peak arousal state.

You might have a fetish for a specific act (such as spanking or bondage), but BDSM is a wider range of behaviors, not a specific fetish.

Kink is a wide term that encompasses so many different acts, but underneath it, each thing shines on its own.

## 5. No "decent" or "good" person would ever be into BDSM

Say it with me now: What happens between consenting adults is completely fine and no one else's business.

Being kinky is not a value judgment. It has no bearing on your worth as a human being.

"The reason many people keep their involvement quiet is because there is still a stigma due to misunderstanding around this practice," Criss tells us. "We don't want to lose our jobs, custody of our children, or any other consequence for consensual activity that is shared with our partners in private." Doctors, lawyers, social workers, school teachers...anyone can be involved in BDSM. Kink is fun.

Kink is not something that needs to be relegated to the shadows. It isn't just for well-seasoned, heavily tattooed babes who wear leather vests and have a penchant for ball gags. It isn't only for the "misfits" of society or people who are "cool" enough to be let into the club. Kink doesn't require that you buy a bespoke corset and various impact play devices to do it "right." It doesn't require you to become a master Dom or sub to engage with it. Kink doesn't discriminate. "Kink combines the physical, emotional, psychological, and spiritual, and it has the potential to heal old wounds," Phillips says. "Kink can deepen connections and relationships, bringing a new level of intimacy, and it can hold a space for creativity, vulnerability, perseverance, control, catharsis, and connection. It is used to cope with anxiety, trauma, depression, and chronic pain."

Kink needs to be normalized.

Kink is simply about sexual self-expression that falls outside of the norm. It is about creativity and exploration of your true, authentic sexual self. It's about following pleasure wherever it takes you. Shame can make this exploration very challenging, even seemingly impossible for some. I want to acknowledge the intense difficulty of this. Shame is a sticky thing. It has a way of seeping into all the crevices of our self-image, wedging its way in and becoming difficult to eradicate.

But I promise that with patience, care, community, and reflection, we can find our way home to our kinky selves. Our kinky selves are inside of us. We just have to be brave enough to find them.

And we're starting this journey together, as a team. Kink is for everyone, and as a card-carrying member of the kink community, I welcome you.

## Chapter 1 recap

In Chapter 1, we endeavored to answer the inaugural question: What even is kink? We looked more closely at kink as a concept and a state of mind rather than just spankings, bondage, and other BDSM activities. When we parse out the deeper intentions behind the practice, we can start to see its benefits in all aspects of life more clearly. Hopefully, you're starting to see that kink is accessible to you, and you can make it whatever you want it to be.

We broke down five common myths and misconceptions about kink, some of which are very much responsible for the negative public perception we have of kink. By unpacking and reframing some of these myths, we can start to unravel shame.

We established that kink is, in fact, for everyone, and no matter who you are, kink is available to you.

Last, we acknowledged shame and the ways this sticky dickhead makes its way into our consciousness—and how it can keep us from exploring our full sexual and erotic potential.

## JOURNAL PROMPTS

1. After reading this first chapter on kink, what kinds of emotions, feelings, or thoughts came up for you?

2. Start to consider what you're hoping to gain from this book and your journey into kink. List three of your goals and reflect. (Examples: to embrace a certain kink, to learn more about a kink, to bring a partner into a kink you have, etc.)

3. Consider your feelings about kink (or maybe the kink(s) you have, or suspect you have)—specifically, consider any negative messages you've received or feelings of shame or guilt that have come as a result of your sexual interests. As we begin this journey, take time to continuously reflect on how these feelings change or progress.

# 2

# POWERPLAY

## The Foundational Layer of Kink Play

**What you'll find in this chapter:**

➔ What is powerplay, and why are people into it?

➔ Powerplay.

➔ Dom/sub dynamic in BDSM.

➔ Top/bottom dynamic.

➔ Vers.

➔ Other forms of powerplay: Caregiver/little, Pet Owner/pet, Tamer/brat.

T o fully understand and embrace kink, we first have to understand power exchange: what it is, why people are into it, and how to do it in a safe and contained way.

Consensual power exchange is the base ingredient of kink play. You can think of it a bit like flour in conventional baking: Without it, you can't bake anything. The same is true for power exchange—you need it, on some level, for a kink scene to transpire.

When I asked Emme Witt-Eden, a former professional Dominatrix and kink expert, how she'd define power exchange, she told me that "consensual power exchange can be defined as the practice of enthusiastically agreeing to either take or give up power when the other participant has also enthusiastically agreed to play this way." It's about two people choosing to occupy roles where power is freely given and taken.

Consent is paramount in this exchange of power. Dr. Nazanin Moali, a sex therapist and the host of the Sexology podcast, says that "since consent is the cornerstone of [kink] practices, it provides an opportunity to ensure the person surrendering control and the person in charge stay within the sexual boundaries they've set."

Witt-Eden points out that without consent, there is no power exchange at all. "When power is taken non-consensually, it's coercion, assault, or rape." No true power exchange happens when both people aren't willingly giving or receiving it.

Power exchange is crucial in kink play for two reasons:

1. It provides the foundational layer allowing the play to take place. One partner willingly agrees to give power to the other for a scene to unfold. Each person has a role that they are playing, with specific actions involved in said role.

2. Consensual power exchange provides a framework for

communication. In this exchange, all partners agree on what's going to happen and communicate their boundaries. Witt-Eden points out that this component is crucial, as people have different ideas of what constitutes a kink scene. Everyone needs to be on the same page.

3.  The specificity of kink scenes and play requires consensual power exchange to manifest in a way that works for everyone. "Just because someone likes being whipped and being humiliated verbally doesn't mean they enjoy cock and ball torture," Witt-Eden says. "Desires are very particular, so it's important to discuss them before engaging in them and agree on what is being practiced in the scene."

There are many different power exchange relationships in kink—and we need to understand the nuances in these dynamics to better understand both kink and ourselves. People often equate kink with D/s (Dominant/submissive) play, but this is simply the most prevalent example of a power exchange relationship. Dr. Celina Criss told me in an interview that language is important when we're talking about these relationships. "I think the distinction of D/s is in the flavor or in how the participants choose to describe what they are doing," she says. "The way we name our identities and activities is part of how we own and experience them. For many, D/s not only indicates a power dynamic but a relationship that might not be present in a power exchange scene."

Criss points to a few examples where power exchange is present, but often without a D/s dynamic.

•   A gang bang or kidnapping scenario could include several empowered participants "taking down" one (or a few participants) who have minimal power. These might be arranged by a Dominant for their submissive and managed by the Dominant, but the D/s relationship doesn't necessarily extend to all participants outside of that event.

- An imperial orgy, or [insert your historical or fantasy theme]. In this instance, a submissive might band together with others to create a total worship experience for their Dominant(s), in which multiple participants tend to the needs and desires of one or a few empowered individuals.

There's definitely a power exchange happening in these kinky scenes, but it isn't necessarily a D/s exchange. What it comes down to is how each person in the scene views themselves, their partner, the play, and the power exchange taking place. Witt-Eden uses the example of a masochist. They may enjoy pain play and torture play, but don't consider themselves submissive. They may view themselves as equal to the person inflicting the pain. It's truly all in the eye of the beholder.

Why are people so horny for power exchange? Let's break it down.

1. Giving or taking control can be exhilarating. Some Doms may enjoy having power if they often experience powerlessness in real life. Subs may have a ton of responsibility in real life and enjoy the surrender that comes with power exchange.

2. For some kinksters, they experience a "flow state" or meditative state when engaged in a kink scene. This is sometimes referred to as "sub space" or "Dom space."

3. The ability to regain a sense of control after trauma can be a big appeal. If you've experienced a loss of agency or control in the past, the power exchange kink can be very healing. We'll get deeper into this concept in Chapter 8.

4. It's highly taboo. This can be especially true when we take gender dynamics into consideration. For instance, a cisgender man giving up power to a woman is not socially acceptable and, therefore, it can be highly arousing.

5. It's just really, really, really hot to play with power. Plain and simple.

This list isn't exhaustive. The reasons for one's interest in power exchange are deeply personal—and something to think about, friend.

Now that we've broken down what power exchange is, let's delve into some of the more specific dynamics that exist in kink—and how they work.

## THE DOM/SUB DYNAMIC IN BDSM AND KINK

While power exchange exists in all kink play, when we're talking about BDSM specifically, the D/s dynamic comes into clear view. "Dominance and submission is the general container for almost all kinks," explains kink instructor and Shibari superstar, Julieta Chiara. This may also be the dynamic you've heard the most about, à la movies like *Fifty Shades of Grey* (which sucks at showing conscious, consensual kink), *Secretary* (which doesn't suck at all), or *Belle de Jour* (also pretty great).

If you're looking to authentically explore kink, understanding what D/s means, how it works, and how to negotiate it in your relationships is foundational. It's essentially the framework that BDSM builds on. Once you understand how D/s dynamics operate, everything else—from floggers and chains to sensory play, fake (or real) blood, or even Jell-O scenes—can layer in more meaningfully.

## What is a Dom?

A Dom is the partner who is calling the shots, so to speak. They are the ones doing the "doing." The way a Dom presents will vary greatly depending on the play and scene in which they are engaging—and personal preference. Criss says that "typically the Dom manages the scene. They might decide things about what the sub wears or how they are expected to behave. They are often, but not always, the 'Top' or 'active' partner—the one using the flogger or giving intense sensations." The Dom's most important role is keeping the sub safe. "They hold their sub in safety throughout the scene," Criss says. "[They tune] in to responses, making sure that boundaries are respected, and accepting the submission as an addition that increases their own power."

Dr. Justin Lehmiller, Kinsey Institute research fellow and host of the Sex and Psychology Podcast, told me in an interview that "the Dom's job is to be assertive, but to do so in a way that is respectful of the trust and boundaries of the sub. It's not a license to do whatever you want without care or concern for the well-being of the other."

## What is a sub?

The sub is the person having things done to them. The sub surrenders power to their Dom and accepts the instruction, rules, and/or sensations provided by their Dom. "Typically, a sub wants to please their Dom," Criss tells me. "Subs who have tasks (boot polishing, service, etc.) will often practice to achieve perfection. When bondage is involved, subs might warm up before a scene by stretching to make sure they are flexible and able to hold stressful positions."

A few examples of subs in BDSM:

**Masochist:** Someone who enjoys having pain inflicted on them.

**Baby girl/baby boy:** Usually enjoys being treated gently and with care. This is part of a Daddy/Mommy/Caregiver/little, Dom/sub dynamic.

**Good girl/good boy:** A submissive who gets off on pleasing their Dom and following orders (essentially the exact opposite of a brat—we'll learn all about brats later).

**Slave:** A submissive who is the servant to their Dom. This dynamic can include sex, but it doesn't have to be sexual. Some consensual slaves enjoy being completely at the disposal of their Dom, with no sex involved.

### What is a switch?

A switch has a very special place in BDSM and kink. These are folx who like to be both a Dom and a sub. This is usually dependent on the context of the scene and/or the partner they are playing with.

For example, a switch may enjoy throwing on leather

high-heeled boots and stepping on one partner in the Dommiest of Dom fashions, but with a different partner, they put on a baby doll dress and sit in their Dom's lap for pets and words of affirmation.

Basically, they enjoy being Dom and they enjoy being sub—it all depends on how they're feeling, what scene is being offered, and who they are playing with.

A switch may also have a strong preference for being a sub or Dom, but is willing to occasionally swap to the other role in the right circumstances. Every single switch is unique and prefers different things.

## WHAT THE DOM/SUB DYNAMIC IS

The D/s dynamic is the context that is built between the Dominant and submissive. It is how they play and relate to one another.

The key word here is "consent." Kink is all about giving and taking power in an empowered way. It's quite a popular saying in kink that "the sub actually has all the control," but this isn't really what is going on here. Yes, the sub certainly has control, but as Chiara points out, everyone in the scene has all the control. It's a mutual exchange between partners, and no one has more control than the other.

Now, here's a real kicker: While Dom/sub dynamics are primarily found in kink, they play out in many forms of sex. One person is usually the more submissive partner, while the other is more dominant. It's within the context of BDSM that we make these dynamics explicit.

## HOW D/S SHOWS UP IN BDSM PLAY

Power exchange shows up in nearly every BDSM scene, but how it manifests can vary wildly. That's part of what makes it so delicious—there's no one-size-fits-all template.

Examples of common Dom/sub relationships:

* Classic Dominance and submission: The Dom commands, disciplines, or directs. The sub submits. It might involve bondage, spanking, punishment, or sensory deprivation.

* Caretaker/little: A nurturing Dom and a submissive in a more childlike, soft role. It's often centered around emotional safety and comfort.

* Brat and Dom: The sub intentionally misbehaves or disobeys to provoke a reaction or punishment. This is a playful dynamic full of tension and push-pull energy.

* Master/pet: A Dom acts as a pet owner, and the sub takes on an animal role—this can include obedience, training, and different forms of animal-centric play.

This list barely scratches the surface, but it gives you a sense of how creative and personal kink can be.

Many people assume D/s scenes are all about physical intensity or pain—but it's so much more than that. As Chiara explains, things like bondage or flogging aren't just about sensation—they're about deepening intimacy and reinforcing trust. "A Dom may consensually practice bondage with their submissive to deepen their power practice," she explains. "Bondage in this scenario can be used as a punishment, a reward, or a sensory experience to show who's boss in a safe way."

## NEGOTIATING BOUNDARIES WITHIN A DOM/SUB DYNAMIC

BDSM and kink are all about negotiation. "Negotiation, or the discussion you have before play, is the place to express boundaries you both have, expectations, and set the stage for consent," Chiara explains. "This helps create healthy boundaries without mystery before entering a dynamic."

The sub isn't helpless or under coercion. Offering power to a Dom is one of the most intimate and empowered choices a submissive can make. The Dom, in turn, accepts that responsibility with intentionality and care.

That's why safe words and ongoing communication are essential. Moali says that "while you should be sure you have a 'safe word' that you may use during the scene to immediately halt any actions, it is [also] important to have periodic conversations about your boundaries." This means checking in to make sure everyone is enjoying themselves and feels safe. Especially when you're new to BDSM, discovering your boundaries takes time. You need to feel safe enough to explore, but also to stop and recalibrate if something doesn't feel right.

And let's not forget that the Dom holds a huge responsibility. They're not just there to lead—they're there to protect. If someone you want to play with tries to skip negotiation and jump into play, it's a major concern.

Chiara says that you *need* to have these conversations. "If someone asks to play before setting any sort of negotiation and boundaries, [that's a] red flag," she explains.

At its core, the D/s dynamic invites us to explore intimacy, trust, and identity in new ways. It's not just about role-play—it's a mirror that reflects who we are, how we relate, and what lights us up.

When practiced consciously and consensually, D/s dynamics

can be one of the most emotionally rich and erotically satisfying ways to connect. There's something incredibly powerful—and beautiful—about giving someone your trust and holding theirs in return.

## OTHER FORMS OF POWERPLAY: CARETAKER/ LITTLE, PET OWNER/PET, BRAT TAMER/BRAT

Now that we've broken down how the D/s dynamic works, let's take a closer look at how the dynamic can exist in different kinds of D/s relationships. Namely, we'll be exploring caretaking dynamics, pet/Pet Owner, brat/Brat Tamer.

Of course, these aren't the only other kinds of dynamics that can happen in kink, but they are some of the most common ones that people tend to explore.

It's important to take a closer look at how some of these Dom and subs relate to one another so that you can start considering what dynamic might feel appropriate (and hot) for you.

### Caretaker/little dynamics

The Caretaker/little dynamic can come with many iterations, including Daddy Dom/little girl (DD/lg), Adult Baby Diaper Lovers, Teacher/student, Bigs/middles, and much more. All of these dynamics intersect with age play. "The thread that the dynamics share is there is someone who is the younger submissive and someone who is the caregiver," kink educator Emerson Karsh told me in an interview. Let's break it down.

Within age play, D/s partners take on characters of different ages within their Dom/sub dynamic. The Dom is in the "Caregiver" role, and the sub is in the "younger" role. "It can involve power dynamics in the sense of one partner being a nurturing, and possibly disciplinary, adult figure and the other partner expressing a dependent childlike persona, needing care and guidance," Criss explains.

Dr. Lee Phillips, a psychotherapist and certified sex therapist, pointed out in an interview that these dynamics can be a part of role-play, or part of a more general lifestyle wherein littles/middles and Bigs live in their preferred age range 24/7.

And before we go any further, *yes*, this kind of play is normal, and you're not weird for being into it. It's *very* important to emphasize that the people who engage in age play are consenting adults who willingly and freely engage with this kink.

Because this play centers around age, the main dynamics can be parsed out into: Caregiver/baby, Caregiver/little, Caregiver/middle, and Adult Baby Diaper Lovers.

- Caregiver/baby: This is also referred to as Adult Baby Diaper Lovers (ABDL). This is when the Dom acts as a Caregiver and the sub acts like a baby or infant. The sub may wear diapers as a part of this play and use non-verbal communication.

- Caregiver/little: This dynamic is also referred to as a DD/lg relationship (Daddy Dom/little girl) or a Mommy/lg dynamic. The Dom acts in the nurturing/disciplinary role, and the sub complies, taking on the role of a child.

- Caregiver/middle: This is also referred to as a Big/middle dynamic. This is when the Dom is the caregiver and the sub is in a pre-teen role. "Middle" is used to indicate that the middle is playing a role that is a bit older than a "little."

## Why are people into this?

At its core, age play is about the giving and receiving of care.

There are so many aspects of this play that kinksters love about being in a Caretaker/little dynamic. "It is often playful and sweet, incorporating nurturing with discipline or behavioral management, which can be a terrific opportunity to express a variety of kinks (spanking, reward/consequence, humiliation, praise, etc)," Criss says. It's highly customizable, giving kinksters plenty of room to experiment and make scenes their own.

For the submissive, the desire to play in a certain age range isn't about *literally* wanting to be a child or baby. It's about wanting to embrace the innocence and carefree nature of being a little—and the comfort of being cared for by someone else.

Professional kinkster and BDSM expert Mistress Kye tells me that these types of age-players may be accessing and regressing to a place of escapism within a simpler time of their lives. "It's understandable why in today's over-stimulated, hectic, and noisy life we all lead, littles and middles play is growing in popularity by leaps and bounds," she says.

For Mommys/Daddys/Bigs/Caregivers, Phillips says the play can offer catharsis on a truly deep level. "Mommy and Daddy types report they enjoy being dominant and caring for others," he says.

Plus, Criss says there is an edginess to it that can be super hot. "It deliberately plays with taboos around age and power dynamics," she says. We love some good old taboo sex.

The point here is that everyone within the dynamic gets what they want out of it.

There are lots of ways that these scenes can play out, and the types of play will vary widely. With that being said, Karsh says the activities people engage with are usually tied to bringing back or creating specific childhood memories. This can include playing with a toy you never received as a child (or one you miss), playing with coloring books, doing puzzles, watching cartoons, etc.

Something I have to bring up again, because it is very import-ant, is that not all kink involves sex. And the same goes for age play. Sometimes it's simply about creating the Big/little dynamic and engaging within these roles.

Now that's not to say people can't find it sexy or that sex can't be involved. Sometimes it can involve specific sexual play and interests, such as punishments and discipline. The activities can be whatever you want them to be. Age play is about the roles you take on in the dynamic, not the specific actions.

## Pet Owner/pet dynamic

Pet play is what it says on the tin, folx. The submissive partner is a pet, and the Dom acts as their Master/Owner/Handler. "It usually involves one or more people adopting the persona of an animal, such as a puppy, cat, or pony," says sex columnist Zachary Zane, author of *Boyslut: A Memoir and Manifesto*. There are endless animal personas people can choose to play—it's all about what each person finds appealing.

Pet play can be scene-specific, as in, it only happens when partners are playing these roles in the context of an agreed-upon D/s scene, or it can be 24/7, where Pet Owners and their pets stay in character all the time. All D/s dynamics can be done in a 24/7 manner, if the partners choose. This might sound a bit intense, but hey, we're not here to judge others—only to learn.

## Pet play in the wild

Rea Pearson, a relationship therapist and clinical sexologist specializing in gender, sexuality, and relationship diversities, told me in an interview that pet play doesn't always require the watchful eye of a Dom. "The owner isn't always a necessary element, as pets can play together without supervision, and sometimes one pet will lead a larger pack of animals," she says. "If a pet doesn't have an owner, they will often refer to themselves as a stray."

While anyone can engage in pet play, Zane says that it is quite popular among the MLM community. "It's common for gay males to have 'pups' who wear dog masks. Their owner or 'handler' may walk them around on their leash while on all fours," he says. "The pup may eat food out of a bowl. When he's being a 'good boy,' the handler may rub his head or give him a belly scratch."

Pet play can also happen in groups, which honestly sounds so fun if you ask me. Zane says these group meetups are called "moshes" and it's "where a bunch of pups get together to roll around, wrestle, and play with one another; the way you might take your (real) dog to the dog park."

## Why do people love pet play

If you've heard of furries, where people dress up in full-on animal costumes, this is a part of pet play. Peason says, "Part of the fun of pet play is dressing up. This can range from something as small as a pet collar, bell, ears, tail, mask, or harness, all the way through to entire anthropomorphic fursuits costing thousands," she says. "The latter are particularly popular with furries, who are pets with entire 'fursonas.'"

If you enjoy pet play, you might like being nurtured and cared for, being used, and humiliated, being punished when you're a bad boy/bad girl, or being rewarded for being good. The reasons someone will love being a pet/Pet Owner are endless and highly individualized. "Some might just want comfort and nurturing, via hugs, belly rubs, tickling, and being fed treats," Pearson explains. "Other pets want to be treated much more roughly or be used for sex, while others have no interest in sexual play and might identify as asexual."

Of course, there is some hot kinky sex in there, too, Zane says. "You can have very primal and animalistic sex when acting as an animal. Some anonymity comes if you or the pet is wearing a mask."

Pet play is a chance to step away from your role as a human being, in which you might be bogged down with responsibilities and anxieties. It's a way to fully embrace joy, even if just for a little while.

### Brat/ Brat Tamer dynamic

Make me, why don't you?

If brats had a signature line, this would be it. "Brats enjoy questioning dominance, and like dominance to be proven to them," says Karsh.

Outside the kink world, being called a "brat" might not go over so well. You'd probably roll your eyes and walk away. But in BDSM, it's a completely different story. A brat is a playful, deliberate role taken on by a submissive who thrives on being rebellious. The goal? To poke the Dominant and get a reaction—one that often leads to a bit of well-deserved (and well-negotiated) punishment. Cue the smirk.

Not gonna lie—this might be one of my favorite D/s dynamics. I know it's hard to pick a front-runner, but there's just something irresistibly satisfying about being a charming little menace.

Mischief, sass, disobedience—it's sexy, it's fun, and it brings an element of levity to erotic play. It's a way to explore your submissive side without falling into the more traditional, obedient mold. Brats are full of attitude, a bit unruly, and often delight in getting exactly what they asked for: trouble.

BDSM is incredibly versatile, and the brat/Brat Tamer relationship is a perfect example of how creative these dynamics can be. "Brats get great enjoyment from playing [a game of] cat and mouse, defying authority, and in turn receiving a 'punishment' from their Brat Tamer," says Chiara.

If playful defiance turns you on, this might call to you. And if you're not sure yet, don't worry. That's exactly what exploration is for.

### So what's a brat?

At its core, being a brat is a sassy twist on submission. It's a persona that's more about playful rebellion than quiet compliance.

Brats don't follow orders just because they're given. They'll tease, test, and stir the pot—usually in hopes of triggering a reaction (and maybe a punishment or two). It's all about pushing boundaries in a way that's fun, naughty, and consensual.

Chiara puts it well: "The brat may taunt, push boundaries, and really test their partner's limits in the hope of causing a reaction. This is very playful, and can be adjusted to your needs."

And yes, it might seem counterintuitive—how can you be both submissive and defiant? But Karsh breaks it down: "Brats express their submission in a way that is amusing, consensual, and done for a reaction." Eventually, the brat will submit—but only after a bit of troublemaking first. And honestly? That's half the thrill.

### Enter: The Brat Tamer

The Brat Tamer is the Dominant counterpart to this dynamic. Whether they go by Sir, Mistress, Daddy, Mommy, or something else, their style is all about reining in that brat energy with confidence and control.

"Their 'role' is to put their brat in their place, remind them of the rules, and enforce the punishments/order that they have created together," Chiara explains. "This is an authority role, and a Brat Tamer must be comfortable with taking control and being taunted by their bratty partner." An example might be a brat playing the role of a defiant assistant to a strict boss.

And make no mistake—this isn't a soft or passive role. Karsh tells us that the brat is not afraid to put their foot down when they need to do so.

But good taming goes beyond dealing out punishments. Karsh adds:

> A brat tamer is skilled in giving their brat space to be a brat and figuring out how to express and prove their dominance to their brat in response to their bratting—whether that be a punishment, orders, ignoring the behavior, or something else.

And yes, everything here is rooted in enthusiastic, ongoing consent. Everyone involved knows the rules, the limits, and tries their best to stay attuned to one another's needs.

### How brats do their thing

There's no one right way to brat—but here are some common approaches that keep things fiery.

### Bratty talk

Verbal defiance is a brat's favorite weapon. Some signature phrases might sound like:

Make me.

That's all you've got?

You wish.

You don't scare me.

What are you gonna do about it?

Oh, please—try harder.

According to Phillips, brats also love pushing buttons through snarky comebacks, refusing instructions, mock tantrums, or interrupting when they're supposed to stay silent. It's all about keeping things playful—and just a little maddening.

### Bratty antics

Behavior-wise, brats love pushing limits in creative ways. Maybe the Dom says, "Get over here," and the brat flops on the floor in protest. Or they're told to be home by a certain hour, and they purposely roll in late with a smirk. It's intentional disobedience with an edge.

And you know what comes next...

When a brat has been naughty, there's usually a price to pay—one they might enjoy just as much as the mischief itself. Of course, every consequence is thoroughly discussed ahead of time. Everyone knows what's in play and what's a hard no.

Some commonly enjoyed "punishments" include:

- spanking

- denial of release

- forced silence

- forced orgasm

- rope play and/or restraint

- tickle torment

- containment (like a cage or being put in a corner).

But here's the key: Punishment isn't a requirement. Not every brat dynamic includes consequences. Kink is customizable—this is your sandbox, and you get to decide what feels good.

Maybe your Dom tames you by holding you down and making you unravel with pleasure. Or maybe they just smile knowingly after you act out, kiss your forehead, and call you a "good little menace." Who says taming can't be tender?

There's no formula here. There's no single "right" way to play. Your dynamic is yours to shape—and that's the beauty of it all.

## The Top/bottom dynamic

In these dynamics, there is still power exchange, but it isn't the same flavor as D/s. Rather, a person is doing and a person is receiving—or a Top and a bottom.

When considering the Top/bottom dynamic, we have to consider the queer community. Topping/bottoming is the way a lot of queer kinky folx think about kink—and sex in general.

A person may be a Top, but they wouldn't consider themselves a "Dom" per se.

Sure, queer folx also indulge in plenty of D/s play, too—but the Top/bottom kink relationship is strongly associated with queer kink. We'll get more into the meat of how Top/bottom dynamics exist within queer relationships and their importance in Chapter 5.

For now, we'll explore a bit of what these dynamics are and how people engage within them as part of their preferred identities during sex and kink.

OK, let's talk about bottoming and Topping.

### Bottoming and Topping

Being a bottom or Top are both very versatile labels.

Dr. Evan Goldstein, a nationally renowned anal surgeon, founder/CEO of Bespoke Surgical, co-founder of Future Method, and author of *Butt Seriously: The Definitive Guide to Anal Health, Pleasure, and Everything In Between*, told me in an interview that "Bottoming holds many different definitions for many different people, but the common thread is being on the receiving end of sexual play. You are the person having things 'done' to you as the bottom partner."

As a Top, you're the one giving sexual play. You are the person doing the "doing." You aren't necessarily in a psychological or physical power exchange dynamic; you're in control of the specific acts taking place.

Here's the thing: Being a Top or bottom isn't all about receiving/giving an object (be it a penis, dildo, etc.) into your holes. These roles are about the *mindset*. Being a Top or bottom is a way of *being* during sex. It is your role—and that can be all-encompassing when in the throes of passion or kink.

Being in your preferred role is an art. It is a skillset. It is a craft.

And as with all crafts, it needs to be perfected with practice and patience. Lying on the bed, receiving from your partner, accompanied by the occasional whimper, is simply not going to cut it—not if you want to be a truly legendary bottom. Standing there and pumping someone into oblivion is not the gold standard Top behavior you want to be engaging in, friend.

Goldstein points out that being a fantastic bottom does not mean giving up full control. The best bottoms can fully embrace their role while retaining control throughout the sex or scene. To do this, he says, "It's imperative to set the stage for success." And in that same vein, much like what we covered with Doms and subs, the Top is not here forcing anyone to do anything. Everyone is an active participant.

### Tops and bottoms in the wild

In the classic sense, a bottom is the receiver during anal penetration. This term is often associated with the gay male and queer communities (MLM). The Top does the penetrating and the bottom is being penetrated. "For gay men, bottoming isn't just a sexual role, it's a lifestyle. That's why many say, 'I *am* a bottom' and not, 'I prefer to bottom,'" explains Zane.

Bottoming has a special meaning in kink play. The bottom is typically the person having things "done" to them. "If you're getting spanked and called a good girl, you may be the bottom in that encounter," Zane explains. The Top is Daddy—the one being served and directing the scene.

In the context of kink, the bottom is usually the submissive partner, but not always. In both anal sex and kink, bottoming and Topping can be deeper than a simple preference. It is a way of sexually and intimately relating.

### Being a bottom vs. being a submissive – being a Top vs. being a Dominant: What's the difference?

Being a bottom and being a submissive are often the same, but they aren't always—especially when we're talking anal sex. While we often use "bottom" and "submissive" interchangeably, a lot of the time, there are key differences. "In reality, someone can be a total bottom and yet be the dominant one in full control," Goldstein says.

This means you may be the one being penetrated, but you aren't the submissive partner. You are the one calling the shots. Your role as the dominant partner is not dictated by whether or not your butt hole is being penetrated. It's all about that juicy *mindset* and the role you're embodying.

It's important to understand this difference—especially at the beginning of your bottoming or Topping journey—because you want to "set yourself up for success," Goldstein adds. You want to get clear about what being a bottom or Top means to *you* and how you want it to look.

### Why bottoms love to bottom and why Tops love to Top

While the reasons someone might find bottoming or Topping enticing (humans are, after all, incredibly varied and complex), the three main reasons appear to be:

1. that receptive anal is very physically pleasurable—for everyone involved

2. the psychological mindset of being a bottom or Top

3. the power dynamics in kink play.

The anus is a hotbed of pleasure. Goldstein says that anyone can unlock the power of an anal orgasm, regardless of gender. And, once you do, it's hard to turn back. "We have many nerve endings that provide pleasure in the anal areas, both internally and externally," he says. "Licking (analingus), rubbing, fucking, fisting—you name it, it stimulates those nerve endings from the entrance all the way up and into the rectum." Plus, you can stimulate the prostate for penis-owners and reach the A-spot through the vaginal wall for vagina-owners. It's pretty epic.

For Tops, well, the anus is incredibly tight and feels very, very good to penetrate. It's not exactly neuroscience.

For those who identify as a bottom, the psychological pull of what this identity means is arousing. You're turned on by being penetrated anally. It's highly taboo, which makes it very sexually exciting.

In kink, the bottom is having things done to them. They are essentially being used—and that is pretty dang enticing and hot.

Tops are turned on by their role as a Top—and what it means to give anal penetration, tie their partner up, or otherwise create a scene filled with intensity and pleasure.

## OK, LET'S TALK ABOUT BEING "VERS" FOR A SECOND

It would be bananas not to talk about the third option in power dynamics: being "vers." This means you are both—a Top or a bottom—usually depending on your mood, the kind of play, and the context.

There are two main ways in which being "vers" comes into play:

1. In penetrative sex (usually sex between two men, but not exclusively).

2. In power dynamics (usually referring to kink dynamics—vers is often replaced with the word "switch," but not always).

These two categories may have a crossover, as in sex can come with power dynamics and power dynamics can come with sex.

As you've probably already surmised, being "vers" means you're into being both a Top and a bottom and/or being dominant and submissive. "A vers is a person who can be a switch," Phillips explains. "Therefore, they may enjoy being dominant and submissive. In sex between two men, they may enjoy being penetrated and [also] being the person who penetrates the anus."

Being "vers" doesn't necessarily mean you're 50/50 in terms of preference for Topping or bottoming. Some vers folx break labels down even further into subcategories. You can be a Top/vers or bottom/vers—meaning you're down for being either role, but you have a strong preference for being a Top or bottom. You're flexible, baby!

Flexible labels can help people identify where they fall on the sexual spectrum. There is a lot of variety and a lot of different ways you can exist as a vers person.

The long and short of it is, being "vers" means you're versatile during sex and are willing to take on the more dominant or more submissive role, and/or you enjoy being both a Top or bottom during sex. The only person who gets to decide if you want to call yourself "vers" is you.

## SHIBARI: ROPE TOPS AND BUNNIES

Let's delve into a good example of how a Top may top without being dominant, and a sub may sub without subbing during kink. Nothing nails it quite like rope bondage. Shibari, or Kinbaku, is the art of Japanese rope tying. It is one of the Bs in BDSM—bondage. Kinbaku means "tight binding," and Shibari means "tying." I just want to be clear, that while Shibari is the most popular form of artistic rope bondage, it isn't the only kind of rope bondage there is. Throughout the book, you will see the word Shibari used—this is intended to be a catch-all for play that involves rope bondage, as many people colloquially refer to intricate rope play as "Shibari."

You know the stuff we're talking about here—Shibari is when you see some super hot hottie tied up in really intricate rope patterns. My personal favorites involve suspension, where the bottom is hung from different rigs and suspended into the air like a human chandelier. If you don't know what I'm talking about, Google it really quickly and come back.

The draw of Shibari is almost spiritual. Chiara, who is a certified Kinbaku instructor, says that Shibari's draw is layered. "It's the erotic nature, blend of pleasure and pain or restraint, and the immense connection and trust that is built between the rigger (one tying) and the rope bottom (one getting tied)," she says.

Shibari, when practiced safely and effectively, can be a fantastic way to play with power dynamics, different forms of pleasure (and pain), and surrender. Historically, it has been seen as an art form and a meditative practice.

There are two main roles in Kinbaku: the rigger and the model.

The Japanese word for the rigger is "nawashi," or "rope artist." The model is often referred to as the "bunny" or "rope bunny." These roles often function in the same way as a Dominant and submissive in BDSM. The rigger is the Dom and the bunny is the sub, but not always. Chiara says that the ways the rigger and bunny relate to one another vary depending on what each person wants out of the scene. "In my tying, I like to make our session a collaboration, as I'm not dominant in BDSM spaces," she explains. "I tie designs and prints on a model's body and take them through a sensory experience: This can include pain, pleasure, sensuality, or somatic release."

The bunny may not be the one tying the knots, but it's still a big job. "Shibari pushes you to surrender," Chiara explains. "Building trust, connection, and safety is a huge part from *both* sides, not just the rigger." Not to mention, you have to stay perfectly still while your rigger ties you into intricate positions.

Some folx practice in a more versatile way, shifting the roles in ways that work for them. "There are instances where people like me explore self-tying (tying oneself, also known as self-suspension) or engage in more fluid roles where both partners share the responsibilities of tying and being tied interchangeably," Chiara says.

In this way, a person may be a rigger, but they aren't dominant. And a rope bunny may be being tied, but they aren't submissive. And yes, it can seem a bit confusing and complicated. But the thing is, every single kink experience and role is customizable for the people engaging with it. That's one of the things that makes it so magical. If you want to be a Dom, you can be a Dom. If you want to be the Top but do not consider yourself a Dom, that's fine, too.

Be a Dom. Be a sub. Be a Top. Be a bottom. Do whatever you want!

Throughout this chapter, we have gone into the weeds about powerplay: what it is, what it isn't, and what it looks like. We've ventured into the different powerplay dynamics that exist within kink and put a magnifying glass up to each to unravel their delicious appeal.

I hope you've learned and found some value in these breakdowns—hopefully, you've gleaned a bit of new information about yourself. Or perhaps, at the very least, I've gotten the cogs of that mighty imagination of yours turning.

Don't worry, my kink-curious friend, by the end of this journey, your hand might just be itching for a flogger.

### Chapter 2 recap

In Chapter 2, we dove into the very heart of what makes kink tick: powerplay. We looked at what powerplay is, how it functions, and why people absolutely love it.

We looked at common powerplay dynamics in kink, unpicking the incorrect notion that all powerplay involves Doms and subs. We looked at the D/s dynamic, Tops/bottoms, and identified the switches and vers folx who enjoy playing both roles.

Last, we got sexy and looked more closely at a few ways powerplay plays out in kink scenes: DD/lg, Adult Baby Diaper Lovers, Pet Owner/pet, Caregiver/little.

## JOURNAL PROMPTS

1. As you read more about power dynamics, what stood out to you? Is there anything that sounds particularly appealing? Why or why not?

2. Do you think you might be a Dom or a sub? Could you be both (vers/switch)?

3. There were three examples of D/s dynamics given in the chapter: Caregiver/little, Pet owner/pet, Brat Tamer/brat. Did any of these dynamics strike a chord? Take some time to reflect.

4. Consider the role of a Top or bottom. Do either of these appeal to you? If so, which one? If this isn't your jam, why do you think that is?

# 3

## KINK VS. FETISH

### What you'll find in this chapter:

➜ The difference between kink and fetish, and why it matters.

➜ Where kinks and fetishes come from—two avenues: conditioning or acquired later in life.

➜ How to tell if you have a kink or if it's a fetish.

➜ Five popular kinks and fetishes, based on data.

**O**f all the chapters in Part I, this explainer might be my favorite. It can help you untangle some of the more tender psychological nuances behind your kinky interests. We're going to delve a bit deeper now into kink vs. fetish. Understanding the differences and how they relate to you personally can help you feel more grounded and solid in your desires. And this can help a whole lot with letting go of shame.

Before we delve in, I'd like you to try to remember three things:

1.  Read this chapter with interest, calm, and open curiosity. We're here to learn about ourselves with open minds and hearts.

2.  If you feel shame, disgust, or other negative feelings coming up for you, simply notice them without judgment—acknowledge their presence—and calmly let them pass through you.

3.  Human beings are complicated, imaginative, and filled to the brim with creativity. Remind yourself of this when it comes to sexuality, both in regard to your own and that of others. This can help us tap into empathy, which is a key ingredient when exploring taboo sexual desires.

Kink and fetish often get thrown into the same bucket of "taboo sexual interests." This isn't surprising given our vast misunderstanding of sexual behaviors and interests that don't follow a strict cis-heteronormative script.

Let's clear up some definitions and take a closer look at these two concepts. The more we know, the better we can understand ourselves and our partners. This, in turn, will lead us to better sexual experiences.

Kink vs. fetish: What is the difference? The world needs to know.

1.  "Kink" is a big umbrella term for all non-vanilla sexual behaviors, acts, and desires.

2.  A kink is a specific sexual interest/preference in a non-normative sexual behavior, body part, object, or act.

3.  A fetish is a specific sexual interest in a non-normative sexual behavior, body part, object, or act. This specific thing is a requirement for full sexual arousal.

When it comes to kinks and fetishes, Phillips (whom we've met in previous chapters) explains that "Kinks [are defined] as a sexual taste or arousal for something that lies outside of normative sexual behaviors or desires." A fetish is an arousal for something that lies outside of the normative sexual behaviors or desires *that are required* for sexual satisfaction and/or arousal. "Given these definitions, a fetish is always kink, but a kink is not always a fetish," Phillips adds.

Who even gets to decide what's kinky, you know? Chiara, our beloved kink expert from the previous chapter, says that you're the only one who gets to define your kinks. "A kink can be as simple as a neck kiss or as intense as being locked in a dungeon cage," she says. There's no concrete definition for what is normal, and there certainly isn't any concrete definition for what's considered kinky.

## WHAT DOES IT MEAN TO BE KINKY?

Let's recap some of our knowledge from Chapter 1 because understanding kink provides a basis for understanding fetish. What makes someone "kinky" is hard to define because of the vastness of human sexual expression. Phillips tells us that kink is "best defined as sexual behaviors and preferences that are not easily categorized or different from what we consider typical sexual interests."

When we say typical, we're talking about "vanilla sex." This refers to sex that would fit into a cis-heteronormative narrative. Phillips says things like the missionary sex position and kissing would fall into the category of "vanilla," whereas kinky sex may involve elements of BDSM, Dom/sub role-play dynamics, leather, spanking, etc.

Kink will usually (not always, but usually) involve elements of BDSM, which focuses on erotic power exchange.

Again, it's not possible to nail down exactly what makes something kinky. Only you get to decide if something is kinky to you.

## SO THEN, WHAT IS A KINK?

A kink is when we have a preference for a "non-normative" sexual behavior or object. We can have lots of different sexual preferences (for instance, we can enjoy doggy style more than missionary), but a "kink" becomes a kink when it isn't typical and doesn't fit into society's conventional understanding of what "normal" sex is.

Since the definition of "typical and normal" sex depends on society, understanding what that even means can be seriously complicated, as we live in a sex-negative world that doesn't like talking openly about sex.

What's important to consider is the word "preference." A kink is a desire for an object or act to be a part of the play. It doesn't need to be there for you to enjoy a sexual encounter, but having it there is preferred. For instance, you may have a leather kink and like it when you and/or your partners dress up in leather during sex. If you don't do this, you can still have a blast doing other things, but it would be great if you could.

## WHAT IS A FETISH?

A fetish is a fixation on a non-normative, typically non-sexual body part, object, or act. A fetish is something a person *needs* to have as part of the sexual experience to achieve full erotic satisfaction.

Some people with fetishes may still be able to have sexual pleasure without the fetish object/present, but many require it to experience sexual arousal and orgasm. "For example, people with a latex or feet fetish may only experience sexual arousal when those [things] are present," Chiara says.

Most fetishes (and kinks, actually) are totally fine to engage with, and anything that happens between consenting adults is OK to play with. As a society, we're deeply steeped in sexual shame, but if we embrace our fetishes in ways that enrich our lives, they can offer fertile ground for exploration. "Body part fetishes are some of the most common fetishes. These can include navels, legs, mouth, and hair. Some people have fetishes with clothing and footwear," Phillips says. "These can include leather, lingerie, gym gear, heels, and other shoes."

Certain fetishes can lead to behavior that is illegal, dangerous, and unethical, Moushumi Ghose, MFT, a licensed sex therapist, told me in an interview. Having a fetish for voyeurism, for instance, can be problematic because watching people have sex without their consent is illegal. There are ways to engage with fetishes safely, but that means playing with them in ways that don't encroach on someone's autonomy or break the law.

## WHY KNOWING THE DIFFERENCE MATTERS

The main difference between a kink and a fetish comes down to the level of intensity. Knowing the difference between whether you have a kink or a fetish "matters because kinks and fetishes come with wildly different sets of standards and needs," Chiara adds.

Kinks = preferences.

Fetishes = requirements.

"There is some crossover between kinks and fetishes—for example, a foot fetish may just be someone's kink in that they love feet, or they love fishnet stockings on feet. But do they need it, absolutely need it, to orgasm? That would be the difference between a kink and a fetish," Ghose says.

Getting clear on definitions matters because it helps us understand our relationship to our specific desires. While most people don't care about definitions in the bedroom, the difference between a kink and a fetish matters for how you approach these acts in your sex life and personal relationships. Think about it for a sec: A partner is probably going to want to know if wearing high heels during sex is something they need to do on occasion for your enjoyment, or if this is something you'll need *all* the time. It helps us figure out our boundaries and what we are or are not willing to engage with.

If the object or act is necessary, it's a fetish. If it's optional, it's a kink. Knowing the difference allows you to communicate more clearly so that you and your partner can co-create a plan for your sex life moving forward.

## WHERE DO KINKS AND FETISHES COME FROM?

There have been two main schools of thought about how sexual preferences primarily develop: social conditioning and genetic inheritance. Fetishes are now widely considered to be developed through conditioning. "Fetishes typically form because we see something that is arousing associated with that object," Ghose says.

For instance, someone with a foot and stocking fetish may find she became highly enamored with stockings and shoes when she was five, stealing them from her parents' friends and hiding them in her room. She may not have associated it with being anything sexual at first, but soon realized that the stockings produced a sexual charge or excited feeling in her body. This sexual charge associated with stockings then followed her into adulthood. And now, here she is, with a stocking fetish.

You may also develop a fetish or kink through "classical or Pavlovian conditioning, in which something that was previously neutral, such as feet, becomes arousing through repeated pairings with sexual activity," says Dr. Justin Lehmiller, a research fellow at The Kinsey Institute and host of the Sex and Psychology Podcast. This means you begin to associate feet (and/or feet-adjacent items) with sexual arousal, after prolonged and repeated exposure.

Additionally, a fetish can develop out of a genuine love of a certain object/body part in adulthood. A perfectly healthy foot fetish can be born out of someone finding joy and arousal in having their feet rubbed or played with as an adult. And suddenly, they have a thing for feet.

Hey, it happens. Humans are wild like that.

And yes, kinks and fetishes are perfectly normal and healthy. We're creative, us humans. It should only be assumed we're going to have creative sexual imaginations.

## SOME HELPFUL GUIDANCE IN TALKING TO A
## PARTNER ABOUT YOUR KINKS AND/OR FETISHES

In Part III, we get very deep into the idea of integrating kink with your actual life and relationships, but while we're on the subject of fetishes, let's look at how we might start thinking about broaching these conversations with partners.

Open and honest communication is absolutely necessary for having fruitful conversations with your partner. It's perfectly normal to be nervous and scared. It's a very vulnerable thing to bring to someone. Asking for empathy and acknowledging how hard it is to be forthright about your kinks or fetishes can help set you up for success.

In order to have conversations in a productive manner with our partners, we need to develop our communication skills around discussing sensitive topics. "Going slow, planting seeds, testing the waters and building safety and communication is something that is very helpful when it comes to talking about kinks," Ghose says.

Here are some examples of how you might approach this conversation with a partner:

* Have you ever had any interesting fantasies around sex? I'd love to talk about them with you.

* Our erotic life is really important to me. I'd love it if we could start having some discussions about expanding our play and figuring out what we're both into. Would you be open to that?

* Would you be open to hearing about something I'm quite interested in sexually? I think it could be a fun conversation. And I'd love to hear your thoughts on fantasy, too!

## WE NEED TO BE CONSCIOUS AND ACCEPTING OF A "NO"

Honestly, your partner might not be down to clown, and we have to accept that. Just because you have a kink or fetish does not mean your partner will definitely be open to engaging with it. This is their right. "That is your partner expressing [that] their interest doesn't match with yours, and that's okay. What isn't okay is to kink shame, or degrade someone for liking what they like. As we say, don't yuck someone's yum," Chiara says.

If a kink or fetish is extremely important to you, and your partner is not currently on board, you have to decide how to proceed. In Part III, you'll have lots of resources and worksheets to plan out these options. Sometimes getting clear on an action plan can help us feel safer and ready to approach difficult topics.

Only you get to decide what this sexual kink or fetish means to you. If it needs to be a part of your life to be happy, it's OK to follow that path. If it's something you don't always need or don't necessarily need, that's OK too.

You're the captain of your ship. Embrace it, baby.

## HAVING A FETISH IS PERFECTLY NORMAL

Let's scream this from the rooftops: There is nothing wrong with having a fetish. There is a ton of stigma and taboo surrounding uncommon sexual behaviors. We feel embarrassed for our "unusual" sexual desires because we've been conditioned to feel shame for wanting to express ourselves in a way that goes against the grain.

There is a need for clear language when discussing these aspects of sexual expression. Having a fetish is a perfectly healthy form of sexual expression. It just happens to be less common than other types of sexual behaviors. Just because something isn't usual or doesn't fit with our socially prescribed views of normality does not make it abnormal, bad, or shameful.

A particular fetish might not be something you see or hear about regularly, but that doesn't make it wrong, gross, or bad.

Having a fetish is perfectly normal as long as you aren't harming anyone else. There can be instances when a fetish can be damaging. For instance, if your fetish were breaking into a person's home and stealing their underwear, this would be extremely problematic. You would be violating their personal space and belongings, stalking, breaking in, and stealing, all of which are illegal. As long as a fetish doesn't break any laws or cause harm to another person or persons, it's fine, and you have no reason to feel ashamed for it.

Whether you have a fetish, know someone who has a fetish, or are simply curious about fetishes, know that there is nothing wrong with you or anyone who has one. Sexuality is fluid, complicated, and mysterious. No matter why something might turn someone on, we have to approach their desire with empathy and without judgment.

## FIVE COMMON FETISHES AND KINKS, BASED ON DATA

### Foot fetishes

Lehmiller's research of over 4175 Americans' sexual fantasies, documented in his book *Tell Me What You Want*, reveals that one in seven people have a foot fetish. According to Google, there are 95,000 global monthly searches on "foot fetish."

"While both men and women can be sexually drawn to feet, men appear much more likely to have this interest than women,"

Lehmiller says. "For example, when I broke my data down by gender identity, 19.5 percent of men said they'd had a sexual fantasy involving feet compared to 8 percent of women."

## Threesomes

According to Lehmiller's data, this is the most popular kink or fantasy. Ninety-five percent of men and 87 percent of women in his study said that they had fantasized about sex with multiple partners.

## Voyeurism

According to a study from Lehmiller's research, voyeurism is very common. In the US, voyeurism has a prevalence of 64.6 percent among men and 34.1 percent among women.

## Bondage

According to a survey conducted by lifestyle website AskMen, 32 percent of respondents expressed an interest in bondage. According to a 2014 study in the *Journal of Sexual Medicine*, BDSM is a wildly common fantasy among people of all genders.

## Public sex

Sixty-six percent of men and 57 percent of women have fantasized about having sex in a public place. Eighty-two percent of both cisgender men and women have fantasized about having sex in an "unusual" place. Think in a car, on a beach, etc.

I'm only providing these five kinks as a way to show you that plenty of people have these thoughts and fantasies. You're simply not weird for being kinky or having a fetish.

---

### Chapter 3 recap

In Chapter 3, we went deep into the wonderful world of fetish. We broke down what a fetish is, how it differs from a kink, and why understanding the nuances of these concepts is important for self-identification and actualization. We did our darndest to look at fetish without shame, and instead with curiosity and empathy, because having a fetish is not creepy or wrong or bad. It is a normal part of human sexual expression.

We briefly considered how we might talk about fetish with our partners as a way to get the mental cogs turning.

Last, we looked at some of the most common fetishes based on research, because the more we start to break down the shame around taboo topics and normalize them, the less shame we feel.

---

## JOURNAL PROMPTS

1. Consider a sexual fantasy you've had and reflect on it. What stands out to you? What happens in your body when you think about this fantasy? When did this fantasy first appear for you? What about this fantasy is appealing to you?

2. We've learned quite a bit about fetish in this chapter. What feelings came up for you? Shame? Disgust? Joy? Thrill? Consider some of these reactions and reflect on them.

3.  Is there a particular fetish or kink that you have or think you might have? If we're being straight with ourselves here, it's pretty likely you have some sort of inclination, or you probably wouldn't be reading this book. Consider your feelings about this kink (or kinks) and fantasy. If you can't think of anything, set a timer for two minutes on your phone and simply sit calmly with your thoughts. See if anything emerges.

4.  Consider how you might broach the conversation about a particular kink or fetish with a partner. Write down a list of everything you'd want them to know and understand about: why this is important to you, what you get out of this kink, and how you hope they will be a part of it (if you want them to be a part of it).

# 4

# UNDERSTANDING KINK

## The Psychology of Play

### What you'll find in this chapter:

→ Kink and adult play.

→ The psychological appeal of kink play.

→ A breakdown of different aspects of kink play.

→ BDSM.

→ Impact play.

→ Bondage.

→ Sensory play.

→ Role-play.

→ Niche play (blood play, breeding kink, primal play, balloon fetish, etc.).

**K** **ink is play.** Understanding this idea is very necessary for you to fully embrace this journey and to dispel shame. What do I mean by this?

Kink scenes are specifically designed for partners to inhabit their desired roles, exercise consensual power exchange, and experience sensations and acts that bring them pleasure and happiness. If you think about it, all sexual and sensual activity between consenting adults can be seen in this way. Kink is a way for us to shed the responsibilities, exhaustion, and anxieties of adult life and engage with a more playful side of ourselves. When we're in a scene, we're playing. We're no longer the grown-ass people who have jobs, kids, and finances—we're just two souls, taking on different roles, engaged in something fun simply for the sake of it.

I sometimes refer to this kind of play as adults getting in touch with their inner child, but this often stresses people TF out. You should see the Instagram comments I get when I merely mention the words "inner child" and "sex" in the same sentence. It really triggers people. I extend empathy to these folx, of course. I suppose they think if we're getting in touch with our "inner child," we're somehow sexualizing children or a childhood experience. This is a misunderstanding that deserves clarity because this could not be further from the truth. Your inner child is a part of you as you are right now—it is a slice of your whole self. It is a part that embraces carefree joy and excitement. And it is often one we exile in the name of productivity and "adulthood" in our capitalist society. To be in touch with your inner child as an adult is to embrace joy. And kink is often a beautiful avenue to finding joy when we so desperately need it.

There are so many different contexts in which to play in kink—and every single one of them could be its own book. To begin to unpick our kinky selves, I've purposefully chosen some of the more popular types of play—and the psychological appeal behind each. Hopefully, with these in hand, you'll start to feel more confident about where you'd like to begin in your kink journey.*

Education is the only way we can begin to unravel our desires. You deserve joy.

## BDSM

When we think of "kink," BDSM is the first thing that comes to mind. It's a media darling, and yet still highly misunderstood. "While people may immediately think of leather, latex, and dungeons, BDSM can be, and is, more subtle than you think," says Criss. BDSM requires consent, planning, and a bit of research.

I know I've mentioned this, but *Fifty Shades* is not, I repeat, *is not*, a good blueprint for healthy and ethical BDSM dynamics. It portrays glorified abuse and throws consent rules out the window. Gag. It makes my skin crawl to think that people would see those movies/read those books and think that's how safe and consensual BDSM goes down. Of course, you're here now, so hopefully, you understand this already. Bless you.

BDSM is an acronym that stands for bondage/discipline, Dominance/submission, and sadomasochism. "BDSM encompasses a wide variety of practices involving intentional play with power dynamics and intense sensations," Criss says. "It is often understood to include role play, fetish, and other practices that aren't considered 'typical.'"

---

* Age play (which we covered in the previous chapter) is also a major form of adult play. I've chosen to skip it here since we've already covered the main points.

As we covered in Chapter 1, "typical" usually refers to anything that falls outside of "normative" sex, and with BDSM, the play is anything but normative. BDSM can be physical, emotional, and psychological. *Play can include sex, but it doesn't have to include sex.*

BDSM is a specific kind of play that falls under the larger catch-all umbrella term of kink. Kink can involve a much larger range of activities, whereas BDSM focuses specifically on dynamics within bondage/discipline, Dominance/submission, and sadomasochism.

## How BDSM usually plays out

BDSM relationships involve a Dominant partner(s) and a submissive partner(s). This is known as a D/s relationship, which you're very familiar with by now. The sub willingly and consensually gives up power to the Dom during the play (often referred to as a "scene"). A scene is co-created between the Dom and sub to look any way they want it to look.

BDSM play can look like:

1.  spanking/impact play: using implements and hands to spank/whip/flog your partner, which we'll break down in more detail later on

2.  bondage: the use of ropes, cuffs, and other restraints—more on this later on

3.  discipline: where the Dom disciplines the sub

4.  humiliation: using certain words or behaviors to con sensually degrade the sub

5. worship: where the sub engages in the worship of their Dom

6. sensory play: engaging or restricting the senses to intensify arousal

7. various role-play dynamics (Caregiver/little, Pet Owner/pet, Master/slave, etc.), which you probably remember from the previous chapter.

And much more. It's anything you want to make of it within the realm of consensual power exchange—and that is what makes it so thrilling and fun. "In BDSM, the world is your oyster," says BDSM educator Julieta Chiara.

## Why are people so hot for BDSM?

At its core, BDSM is all about the giving and receiving of control. People are into BDSM for highly personal reasons. When we engage in high-intensity activities like painplay and bondage, our brains release chemicals like dopamine, oxytocin, adrenaline, and cortisol. The rush can be euphoric, explains Ness Cooper, a kink educator, sexologist, and therapist.

Adrenaline is the hormone released when our bodies experience a "fight or flight" response. This happens when our brains and bodies perceive that we are in danger. "Pain and pleasure are closely related and processed in the same parts of the brain, meaning that those [who are] into receiving consensual pain can feel pleasure from these BDSM acts," Cooper says. Studies confirm this. But you may also genuinely find experiencing pain pleasurable, too. Different strokes for different folx.

Cortisol is the body's stress hormone. A 2008 review of two studies found that this hormone was highly elevated for participants who were receiving stimulation, bound, or (consensually) following orders during BDSM play (Sagarin *et al.*, 2008).

What's more, it's about so much more than spankings and chains, y'all. Its appeal can be quite wholesome. "BDSM is about playfulness, expression, and exploration," Criss says. It's an "opportunity to explore your desires and embrace parts of your self-expression that might not have another socially accepted outlet." This can be very liberating. BDSM play offers a place for us to explore our most taboo desires. It's a safe space to enjoy our sexuality and release shame.

Engaging in these activities with your partner(s) fosters intimacy because it's highly vulnerable to consensually give and receive control. It takes a lot of trust, and, possibly most of all, it's fabulous because it's fun.

### Impact play

Let's talk about the art of getting smacked, in a consensual, sexy way. Impact play can involve anything from slapping, spanking, and hitting to more creative forms of physical play.

Impact play "can [involve] hitting, punching, or slapping, but you can also get creative like [being] pummeled with fists, alternating different strokes or slaps," says Lucy Rowett, a certified sex coach and clinical sexologist. Of course, it doesn't have to be all hands-on—you can bring in toys like paddles, floggers, whips, crops, or even get a little resourceful with items from around your home.

Impact play is exactly what it sounds like: using physical contact—whether with hands or tools—to build sexual energy, offer deep sensations, and deepen power exchange in kink dynamics.

Here are some examples of impact play:

- flogging
- paddling
- caning
- spanking (with hands or tools)
- using a crop.

## So...what's the appeal?

From a neurological standpoint, this makes a lot of sense. Pleasure and pain aren't opposites—they're closely linked in the brain. Research shows that both activate overlapping areas of the brain, which explains why some people get turned on by pain. When you experience physical intensity, your nervous system floods you with endorphins—natural chemicals designed to ease pain. That endorphin high can feel euphoric, almost intoxicating.

Some folx are wired to crave this blend of pain and pleasure. People who get aroused by receiving pain are known as masochists, and as we know, that's where the M in BDSM comes from. "Aside from the sensation, [impact play] is a magnificent tool to reinforce kinks/BDSM dynamics like Dom/sub as tools for 'punishment' or 'reward,'" says Chiara.

There is a caveat here that we need to clarify: Not all impact play is pain play. This is where a lot of people get confused. Words like caning or flogging might sound intense, even violent—but impact play doesn't have to be painful, says Criss. "Players will vary their strikes to achieve the desired effect, ranging from soft and gentle to firm to stingy." Whether you're into soft, teasing swats or full-on power smacks, it's all about what works for you and your partner(s). However you enjoy your impact, it's totally valid.

## SAFETY AND CONSENT ARE EVERYTHING

You've heard me say it before, and I'll say it again (and again, and again): Consent is everything, especially when we're talking about striking someone's body during play. You can't mess around with this. Every impact scene needs to be fully discussed and agreed upon beforehand. This isn't something you just spring on someone in the heat of the moment.

Yes, impact play can be super hot, but it also comes with real risks, and it deserves thoughtful preparation. "BDSM players of any type need to understand the risks inherent to the play they want to engage in: physical, mental, and emotional," Criss explains. "Experienced players have typically studied their activity of choice, the anatomy involved, first-aid care for when things go wrong, and are practiced in communicating throughout the play."

Communication is so, so key. "Don't ever attempt to start hitting or striking your partner during play or during sex without communicating beforehand; it can put them into a threat response," Rowett says. It's a serious boundary violation and can be incredibly damaging if done recklessly. And when it comes to safety, it's important to consider joint placement when practicing any form of impact play. You don't want to hit joints during impact play at all (such as the wrist, ankles, shoulders etc.), as this can lead to injury—and even nerve damage. Avoid these areas carefully.

So yes, have fun—have lots of fun—but be informed, intentional, and respectful. We'll go deeper into specific safety techniques in Part II, so you'll be well equipped to do this right.

## BONDAGE

Bondage is possibly the most intensely popular form of kink play. In fact, according to Dr. Justin Lehmiller's survey of over 4000 people about their fantasies, BDSM play is one of the most popular sexual fantasies we have. There's no shame in it. Studies have shown that nearly half of all Americans have tried restraint play in some form or other.

Bondage is that trusty B at the beginning of BDSM. It is the act of restraining or being restrained.

Types of bondage can include:

- Shibari (Japanese rope tying)

- handcuffs

- bondage tape

- using your hands

- silk scarves as restraints (and other household objects)

- harnesses

- cages.

### Why love bondage?

Bondage is an immersive way to surrender control for a submissive partner. They have to lie back, be in their body, and stay in the present moment. It's a profound act of submission and trust.

For the Dom, there is an element of complete control that can be appealing. You're also creating an experience to give another person (and yourself) pleasure—this can be such an amazing way to step out of the anxieties of life and be fully embodied. Tying someone up can be therapeutic and even healing.

For people who love Shibari specifically, it's true artistry. You're taking the time and care to create elaborate rope creations on a sub's body, allowing them to pass into a deeply meditative state.

While people are into bondage for many reasons, it seems to be highly focused on the act of surrender and the bond it creates between play partners. I know this may sound unexpected, but it's actually really intimate for many people who practice it.

## SENSORY PLAY

Let's be clear: Kink isn't just whips and pain—it's about sensation. At its core, kink is a celebration of the senses. As kink educator Criss puts it, "Pain never needs to be involved in sensual sensory play." Criss continues, "Think gentle touches, delicious flavors, delightful scents, different kinds of light, and beautiful soundtracks. The clothes we wear and the settings we create can be a big part of this sort of play."

Sensory play is simply play that engages the senses—touch, smell, taste, sound, and sight. Sure, it can involve pain, but it doesn't have to.

Deliberately engaging the senses to explore pleasure is what sensory play is all about, according to Criss. "This is where we get the word sensual; it can mean nearly anything in a play context," she says.

Chiara says, "You can enjoy pain-free sensory play with things like massaging, tickling, feeding each other fruit, blindfolding, erotic music, etc. They all play a part in[to] a larger, more sensory experience."

It's all about curiosity, creativity, and how power exchange can be expressed through sensation, not necessarily intensity or pain.

In the kink world, we like to say: Don't yuck someone else's yum. However you enjoy your play is valid and beautiful.

## Why sensory play feels so damn good

Every sensory scene is unique—it all depends on what feels good for you and your partner, and the boundaries you've discussed. There's no one-size-fits-all experience.

Here are just a few ways sensory play might look:

- using a blindfold to remove sight and heighten other senses

- covering the body in whipped cream to lick off

- bondage (ropes, cuffs, harnesses, cages, etc.)

- caressing the skin with feathers, silk, or fur

- using temperature play (ice cubes, warm oils, heat packs)

- wearing a hood or mask to block light or sound

- sensual massage

- edging (teasing arousal without orgasm)

- feeding each other fruit or tasting new textures

- playing with sex toys or vibrational sensations

- soft, light spanking or paddling—no pain necessary.

This list isn't exhaustive, but it gives you a good idea of the range and creativity involved. And remember that intensity is optional. "I can't emphasize enough that you don't need to go hard. Light paddling and spanking can go a long way," Zane tells us. "You really,

really do not need to wallop your partner for an enhanced sexual experience." Ultimately, sensory play is about creating connection and deepening intimacy through sensation, exploration, and trust.

Sometimes, sensory play is about enhancing a particular sense. Other times, it's about removing one to heighten the others, "such as using a blindfold so you can't see," says *Boyslut* author Zachary Zane.

### Sensory play: With or without pain?

Here's the thing—pain play is sensory play because you're feeling it through touch. However, not all sensory play involves pain.

Think of sensory play as the big umbrella category, and pain play as one specific piece of it. Some folx enjoy both, some prefer one over the other, and all of it is valid. Sensory play expands beyond just touch—it taps into every sense.

### ROLE-PLAY

Role-play is one of the most accessible kinds of kinky sex. It is where fantasy and reality intersect. This is when you decide to make one of your mind's imaginary scenarios a (somewhat) reality. If you want to act out a fantasy, you can do so.

It's just playing pretend. As long as you're not acting on anything illegal or particularly dangerous, and everyone in the scenario is a consenting adult, you're absolutely welcome to do your thing.

There are a million different ways to role-play; you just have to find what works for you. There is no right or wrong way to participate, as long as you're being safe and conscious of everything and everyone around you.

## Why do we love role-play?

When we role-play, we get to become someone else. You're meta-phorically wearing someone else's skin for the evening.

You and your partner have a chance to step outside of your daily roles and be whoever you want to be. Whether it's a couple from a movie, a football player and cheerleader, a handyperson and a hot housewife—anything is possible when you're role-playing.

It's a safe space where you can let go. You and your partner are not just acting out a fantasy—you're a part of the fantasy.

Dressing up is fun! You have total control over the scene. You can role-play by simply taking on a certain character and talking dirty to each other. But you can also choose to have more elaborate scenes—ones with costumes and gear.

Say, for example, you want to do a college student/professor role-play. You can go to the store and buy a coed-esque outfit and a pair of fake glasses for your partner. Perhaps you even want a riding crop since you've been a bad girl?

Preparing for a scene is a kind of mental foreplay. You're already playing the role before you begin the scene. Buying things for your role-play and setting up the gear is super hot. Touching a leather riding crop, seeing a certain outfit you plan to wear, and imagining all the things your partner will do to you later—it's one giant collective turn-on. You're already thinking about what's to come.

Plus, for couples who aren't into heavy BDSM, but want to keep things hot, novelty can help with that. As anthropologist Dr. Wednesday Martin points out in her book *Untrue*, one of the main things that keeps a spark alive in monogamous relationships is novelty. We have trouble wanting what we already have. Role-play offers that taste of the unknown that we crave. Put simply, it is new. It's something different.

As much as we may not want to admit it, we all fantasize about other people. It's completely normal and healthy. It's one of the beautiful things that makes the wild imagination of human beings so unique. Role-play is a chance to play with those edges.

## NICHE PLAY

The kinds of play we engage with often don't fall strictly into the broader boxes we've outlined so far. More niche forms of kink and fetish play certainly incorporate elements of sensory play, BDSM, and role-play, but they are more highly customized. These forms of play are centered around more specific interests and objects.

Some examples of niche play:

- blood play

- primal play

- breeding kink

- balloon fetish

- sploshing (a sexual fetish for jelly-like, wet, and messy substances)

- foot worship

- macrophilia (giantess kink).

And just so, so, so much more. As I always say to folx who innocently ask me about my job: If you can think it, people will do it.

The reasons people engage with more niche styles of play are highly varied (surprise, surprise!), and so it's impossible to paint with broad strokes when considering the psychology behind their appeal.

To offer a glimpse into why someone might be into more niche play, let's take a look at two examples: breeding kink and blood play.

## BREEDING KINK

This kink eroticizes unprotected sex, either anal or vaginal. This kink, like all kinks, is practiced with full consent from all parties. A breeding kink refers to the intense arousal at the thought of being impregnated or impregnating someone. A breeding kink means you are turned on by the idea of becoming pregnant during sex, or making your partner pregnant.

Your kink is quite literally to breed or be bred. This means wanting someone to ejaculate inside of you—or wanting to ejaculate inside of your partner—either as fantasy or reality. This kink can be practiced by any couple/group of any and all genders.

This kink is popular across the gender spectrum but is particularly popular with the MLM and gay male community. Phillips says that gay men often fantasize about the risk of getting pregnant, even though they can't. They find the fantasy incredibly hot.

What breeding kink can look like, and where it can intersect with other forms of play:

- HuCow (human cow fetish—which is a subset of animal role-play)
- pregnancy kink
- alien implantation fetish.

And more!

## Why do people love breeding kink?

There's a danger and risk element. For some people, it's undoubtedly about the risk involved with unprotected sex and pregnancy, as danger can be a huge turn-on.

Powerplay is a big component, as with all kink play. The D/s dynamic is central to all kink and BDSM play. It's about giving and receiving control. In breeding Dom/sub-type powerplay, one participant is controlling the other to make them pregnant. It's about the taking and giving of total control.

Believe it or not, there is also a connection and bonding that comes from this play. For some breeders, the desire to form a deep and connected emotional and physical connection with their partner could be the main erotic motivator. Being tied to someone for life can form intense, intimate bonds.

## BLOOD PLAY

An interest in blood and sex is not unusual. In Dr. Lehmiller's survey, he found that 17 percent of women and 9.5 percent of men said they'd had fantasies involving blood. Blood fetish, or a blood kink, is when someone is aroused by the sight, smell, scent, taste, and/or look of blood. Blood is a source of sexual arousal.

What blood play can look like and where it can intersect with other forms of play:

- period sex

- doctor role-play

- vampire role-play

- giving or receiving piercings

- intentionally drawing blood (with knives, needles, or surgical equipment).

And more! This kind of play can be quite dangerous when it involves real blood, so safety and caution need to be front and center. Many blood players opt for using fake blood (which you can easily order online) to be able to safely engage in this kink without the risk.

This kind of play incorporates many of the other broader categories we've already broken down, namely, sensation play, BDSM, bondage, and role-play.

## Why do people love blood play?

Blood play is a pretty niche activity within the BDSM community. Cooper, who is a retired pro Dom who specialized in blood play, says that "those into blood play may be a masochist wishing to have blood-letting-style injuries occur on their body." Those who enjoy performing blood-letting activities on their partner may get erotically stimulated by seeing their partner's blood.

As with all BDSM, there is a huge element of powerplay in a lot of bloodplay. For instance, in a doctor role-play scene, the doctor (the Dom) is taking blood from their patient (the sub). Powerplay can be hugely erotic, and erotic pain can be very intense.

For those who enjoy blood play, the benefits include the rush of endorphins and other feel-good chemicals that get you going. There is definitely something very animalistic and primal about blood. It's a fluid that has had poetic weight for centuries.

Cooper says that people who enjoy vampire fantasies often drink each other's blood in an "almost romantic way." The psychology behind the desire to sexually engage with blood is complex.

Long story short: People are into blood play because it's primal, raw, involves powerplay, is bonding, and is mad taboo.

### Chapter 4 recap

Throughout this chapter, we have explored the myriad ways in which adults use kink to explore and play. We've broken down some of the more popular, and a few of the niche, ways that we use imagination, sensation, and creativity to create saucy scenes for pleasure and fulfillment.

We looked at:

- BDSM
- impact play
- bondage
- sensory play
- role-play
- niche play (blood play and breeding kink, specifically).

Last, we broke down some of the reasons *why* people enjoy this stuff. Oftentimes, it just takes looking more closely at the psychological reasons why people enjoy kink to see that it is far from weird, dangerous, or shameful. Much of kink play serves to fulfill longings that we just don't get [to fulfill] in real life. It's a beautiful way to experience joy and bond with other like-minded folx. It's a way to embrace our shadow side and integrate our desires instead of banishing them to the back corners of our minds.

When we let go of shame and embrace our joy, we are suddenly much freer, don't you think?

## JOURNAL PROMPTS

1.   Did any of the broader categories of kink play jump out at you?

2.   Reading through this chapter, what emotions, feelings, or thoughts came up for you?

3.   After reading the section on niche play, did anything come up for you? If you've found your interests to be centered on more specific acts or objects, reflect on *why* you find them appealing.

4.   After reading this chapter, how are you feeling about kink play in general? Has anything shifted for you after reading about these topics in a shame-free way? Reflect on your feelings and anything that might have changed. And if nothing has changed, reflect on that, too!

# 5

# THE INTERSECTIONS OF KINK, QUEERNESS, GENDER DIVERSITY, AND NEURODIVERSITY

## What you'll find in this chapter:

→ How queer and gender-diverse populations find a home in kink.

→ An exploration into how marginalized identities tend to flock toward each other to build community.

→ Bottom/Top/vers meanings and adaptations.

→ Kink as a sexuality.

→ Kink, asexuality, and neurodiversity.

→ How kink can help to explore sexual pleasure and safety after trauma among queer and gender-diverse folx.

→ How kink can help build new pathways to sexual exploration in a gender-affirming way.

→ A look at how kink intersects with open and polyamorous groups.

**W**e cannot talk about kink without talking about queerness, gender diversity, relational diversity, and neurodiversity. They all intersect to such a degree that when I asked Rufai Ajalan (Roo), an intimacy coordinator, about it in an interview, they said that, if it were a Venn diagram, it would just be a circle.

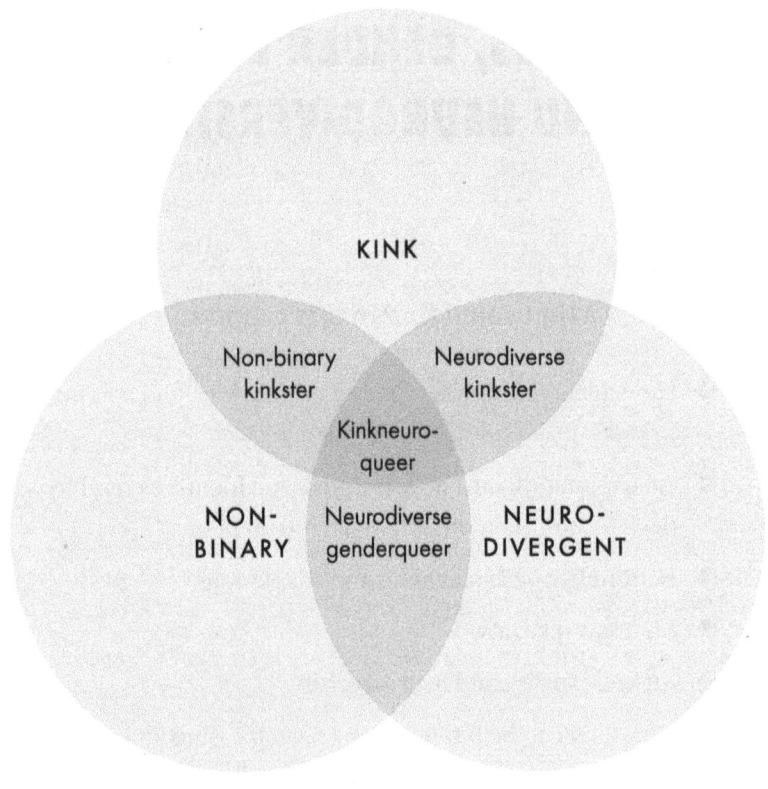

All jest aside, I want to start by making it clear that this chapter is not going to be a "freak show" in which we try to fit all the diverse, non-vanilla, and non-heterosexual populations into one convenient chapter and call it a day. I've been in many a training session where this has been attempted, and let me tell you, it sucks. These topics are far too complex to be boiled down to their respective bones. Rather, this chapter will attempt to introduce very complex topics in a concise way that will hopefully encourage further personal exploration and learning. It will be like dipping a kinky french fry into a giant vat of much more complicated, interdimensional ketchup. It's just a taste. We are going to go over some of the most important intersections with diverse populations and kink because we have to give the hat tip where it is warranted. Kink has its roots in queer and diverse culture, and we should never forget that.

Check out the resource page at the end of the book for more books to read, workshops to take, and documentaries to watch to learn more about these topics. Hopefully, I can do my community justice in the space allotted. And with the help of some of my trusted friends and colleagues within these marginalized groups, I have faith I can.

Buckle up, children! This one is going to be a bit of a ride.

## HOW QUEER AND GENDER-DIVERSE POPULATIONS FIND A HOME IN KINK

Diverse populations have always found a home in kink. The intersection of queerness and kink has a long and rich history. For instance, the "Hanky Code" was first used in the 1970s and 80s as a signal for queer men looking for partners to engage in BDSM. A hanky was placed in the back pocket of the pants as a code to the like-minded. Likewise, the history of leather in the gay male community goes back to the 1940s. It's not new!

Diverse populations find a home in kink for many reasons, but I'd argue that the main reason is the taboo nature of kink.

It is considered to fall outside the norm. Diverse populations already don't fit in with the "normal" or socially prescribed hetero-normative narrative and, therefore, they have a lot more room to experiment with taboo play. Marginalized groups of people tend to flock toward each other to build community. It's a chosen family. "In queer, kinky spaces, we get to embrace the sweetness of community, we get to feel part of a group that really gets us, and we get to explore our fantasies away from prying eyes," explains Poppy Scarlett, a sex and non-monogamy educator. "There is so often a tenderness and a sweetness in these spaces, where queer people hold space for each other's big feelings along with silliness and filth. Queer kinky spaces can feel like a sanctuary."

If you're already not accepted by mainstream society, what's to stop you from enjoying adult play that isn't mainstream? As Leanne Yau, a polyamory educator, sex-positive advocate, and founder of the Polyphilia blog, told me in an interview, it's all about pleasure outside the box: You're already outside the box, so why not just do what brings you pleasure and makes you happy?

As a sex therapist specializing in sexuality and relationship diversity myself, I've always found this enmeshment of kink and queerness to be very comforting. It's a way to bring together folx who feel "othered" and help them find a home while exploring their desires authentically. To me, this is deeply healing. "Kink is a way for people to come into power after being oppressed for so long by a society who seeks to tear us down," Yau adds.

## TOP/BOTTOM/VERS MEANINGS AND ADAPTATIONS

Diverse populations will use the terms Dom and sub in kink, but they may also choose to use Top/bottom/vers, too.

We've covered the meanings of Top, bottom, and vers, but

how do they differ in meaning for queer folx in the realm of kink? Rhi Kemp-Davies, a non-binary psychosexual therapist who specializes in working with trans/non-binary people, says they aren't entirely sure if these terms are always used differently than in cisgender kink relationships, but "gender-diverse people can think and reflect more on what things mean so they may apply more nuance to these words, which means they are more likely to discuss this in every new scenario rather than make any assumptions."

What these terms mean to you may not fall inside of the "prescribed" meanings assigned to them. How you show up as a giving or receiving partner in kink can be entirely personal and inter-relational. Shae Harmon, a non-binary psychosexual therapist who works with the queer community, says that within kink, which is often a subculture of queerness, it's really about the expansiveness of the play. There's just more room for choosing your own kinky adventure and kinky personality when you're already so used to thinking outside of the culturally prescribed box.

To me personally, that's one of the most beautiful things about kink and queerness—there's just so much room for self-expression and personal interpretation. It's not about doing kink "right"—it's about doing kink right *for you.*

And what's more, Poppy Scarlett pointed out to me in an interview that the label someone takes on—whether Top, bottom, vers, Dom, or sub—has absolutely nothing to do with the person's genitals, so this can be very liberating.

## KINK AS A SEXUALITY

For some folx, kink is more than a practice within their sex lives. Some people consider kink a part of their sexuality. For example, a person may identify as gay and kinky. They may also just identify as kinky, with no other label attached to it. Kink is an integral part of their sexuality and identity, and this is valid.

As sex therapist Dr. Lee Phillips puts it:

> For some kinky people, kink can be one small part of their sexuality. For others, it can be the predominant way to enjoy sex. Kink can also be the exclusive way that some people express their sexuality and an integral part of their lifestyle and identity, which improves their overall mental health and self-esteem.

## KINK AND ASEXUALITY

Asexuality falls on a spectrum, ranging from not experiencing sexual attraction at all to experiencing it within certain contexts. For asexual folx—even those who are sex-repulsed—kink can still be a big part of their lives.

You might be wondering: *How is that possible?*

Well, it takes on a different meaning for them. Kink is not about sexual gratification, per se, but about experiencing sensation and/or playing with power dynamics in an authentic way. I put out a call on the socials to ask those in the asexual community why they enjoy kink and received the following responses:

> It's a chance for me to be out of my head and in my body.

> Powerplay isn't always about sex, and that is what kink is for me.

> I can enjoy pain, but it isn't sexual for me. It's about the pain itself.

> Giving up power is a way to experience myself differently.

> I can feel sexy without it being sexual.

Sensation in kink can bring me to orgasm, but it isn't necessarily sexual. It's a release.

I get to play different roles, and that's exciting to me.

Kink isn't sexual to me at all. It's all playful.

## KINK AND NEURODIVERGENCE

Similar things can be said for some neurodiverse folx. As Harmon puts it:

For neurodivergent individuals [it's a way] to explore sensation or sensory physical experiences without it having to do with anyone's genitals. And because it doesn't have to do with genitals, people might have real interest in something like leather, but they don't want that sexual connection. They want that more playful connection or something like that.

For neurodivergent folx, kink has so much to offer because it stands quite outside socially prescribed norms.

What kink can offer neurodivergent folx:

- Sensory stimulation in a controlled way. This can look like deep sensations, sensory deprivation/enhancement, and pain play.

- Less social pressure. When we're playing in kink, social norms around sex essentially go out the window, and we're free to co-create our dynamics, interactions, and actions within a scene.

- Clear communication around boundaries and consent.

Essentially, because kink encompasses so much and can offer people so much expansiveness, there is room for nearly every single person to get something out of it, all customized to fit their exact needs.

## HOW KINK CAN HELP TO EXPLORE SEXUAL PLEASURE AND SAFETY AFTER TRAUMA AMONG QUEER, GENDER-DIVERSE, AND NEURODIVERSE FOLX

Within the queer, gender-diverse, and neurodiverse communities, there are a lot of traumatic experiences that can deeply affect our mental health. This won't apply to every person, but you'd be hard-pressed to find a marginalized person who has not experienced trauma as either an indirect or direct result of their identity. When we experience trauma, we lose a sense of control, and this can be incredibly disempowering.

Kink can be used as a tool to take back control. It's a way for marginalized folx to examine their relationships with power dynamics in a safe and consensual way. Within kink, you get a chance to give up or take power in a way that is empowering. "It's a fantasy world where we can play out power dynamics in exactly the way we desire, we can take autonomy over our bodies and perhaps even re-live emotions and experiences that we previously had no control over," says Poppy Scarlett.

"[Kink is] a way of building trust and forming connections. And that can really be a practice of control and boundaries and consent and negotiation, while also sort of letting emotions flow freely through the body," Harmon says.

Kink and mental health will be expanded upon in Chapter 8, where we'll deep-dive into how kink can be a tool in healing trauma. This can be true for anyone of any identity, but when it comes to gender-diverse populations, it takes on particularly tender significance.

## HOW KINK CAN HELP BUILD NEW PATHWAYS TO SEXUAL EXPLORATION IN A GENDER-AFFIRMING WAY

Kink is a container for such a wide range of play and sexual roles that the ways it can be used are essentially endless. When it comes to exploring your desires in a way that feels gender affirming, it allows you to break outside of gender norms and say "fuck it" to how you're "supposed" to behave. You get to completely rewrite the script in a way that feels good and right for you.

As Kemp-Davies so eloquently put it in an interview:

> A lot of gender-diverse people are much more likely to experience gender dysphoria. Because of this, they can find it more difficult to have sex in a way that the normative sexual script has told us to. As a result of this, when "penis in vagina only" sex causes psychological and physical discomfort, you are more likely to start considering other ways to explore sexual pleasure. When you find yourself in a marginalized gender identity, you are forced outside of that box of normativity, which then gives you space to think about what you want to do, rather than what others expect you to do. This is when kink can help you connect with pleasure and exploration of sensations. Kink opens up a world of play and experimentation, and in a basic sense, it gives a person access to pleasure for the first time, and connects them with their gender more authentically.

The use of fantasy—a cornerstone of kink, as we know—can be incredibly powerful when you're seeking play that feels gender affirming. It's a chance to explore what you desire in a way that feels safe.

For example, role-play can be a powerful tool in exploring your gender identity. "Fantasy is a wonderful way to explore different aspects of your identity, including 'giving it a go' and seeing how it feels without m/any repercussions," says Kemp-Davies. "It's a wonderful experience for a transfemme person to be called a princess or for a transmasc person to be called handsome for the first time!"

Harmon adds that a lot of kink play doesn't include genitals, which can be really healing and helpful for gender-diverse folx, who may experience dysphoric feelings around their genitals.

Sex is about so much more than genitals—and kink is about so much more than sex!

## HOW KINK INTERSECTS WITH OPEN AND POLYAMOROUS GROUPS

As with other marginalized groups, relationally marginalized groups can also find a home in the kink community. There is a huge overlap between those who identify as non-monogamous and kinky. As we've said, those who are marginalized will tend to flock together to find community.

Roo says that they moved into a polyamorous relationship structure as a layered part of their journey into kink. While they say kink wasn't exactly a "gateway drug" into relationship diversity, the experience of being around so many diverse populations and different relationship structures opened up the ability to reflect on how they wanted to live their life. It was an opportunity to explore who they were and what worked best for them within a strong community of support.

Being in a diverse community is not going to "make you

polyamorous" or "make you queer"—but it does open the doors for deeper self-exploration and reflection that can lead to larger revelations about yourself. That isn't something to be scared of; that's something to be celebrated.

"My perspective is that when you openly own one identity that is perceived as 'other,' (queerness, kink, non-monogamy) then it's a lot easier to claim another," says Poppy Scarlett. "You've already done the hard work of reconciling the fact that you perhaps don't fit into the mainstream or you've come out as being part of a vilified group; once you've done this, it can feel a lot easier to own another."

The bottom line: Kink in the real world isn't anything like the heterosexual, *Fifty Shades*-style portrayal we see in mainstream media. The kink community is full of marginalized community members, and kink itself is a marginalized community. It might be full of leather and floggers, and humiliation kinks—but I promise it's one of the most fun and judgment-free places to be on planet Earth.

---

### Chapter 5 recap

Chapter 5 was an overview of the many intersections of kink with marginalized identities, including gender-diverse, relationally diverse, and neurodiverse populations. We briefly touched on where kink falls within these communities and what it means for marginalized folx to practice kink authentically.

---

## JOURNAL PROMPTS

I.   If you could leave expectations around your gender behind, what would your kink practice look like? Would it change? Stay the same? Are there other roles or dynamics you'd want to explore if you knew there would be no judgment?

2.  Where do you see intersections with your identity within marginalized groups (if you do)? What does that mean for you? How might this play into your kink practice?

3.  When it comes to kink, what excites you about it beyond sexual gratification? Is it sensations? Powerplay and consent? Something else? Reflect on what deeper meaning or expansiveness kink might bring to your life with this in mind.

4.  After reading about the interrelatedness of kink with marginalized groups, how do you feel? How might this knowledge impact your practice?

# PART II

# KINK AND SEXUAL HEALTH

# 6

# PHYSICAL SAFETY

## The Basics

---

### What you'll find in this chapter:

→ STI prevention and screening.

→ Vetting potential kink partners.

→ The rules of RACK.

→ Learning your stuff and practicing your craft.

→ Have plans in place if something goes wrong.

→ Exercises.

---

**W**elcome to Part II! Congratulations! You've done a crash course in kink 101, and now you're ready to start learning more of the hands-on tools you need to safely *practice* kink. We're moving away from theory and psychology, and into the nitty-gritty, usable stuff.

Before we start, take a minute to feel proud of yourself. We've covered a *lot* of information in a very short time.

In this chapter on physical safety, we're going to look at a lot of general information that can (and should!) be used for all kink play. We'll also spend some time looking at more specific types of play, particularly play that involves more risk, such as bondage and impact play. We really do need to know how to do these activities safely to avoid injury.

I want to offer a disclaimer before we dive in: This guide is not a replacement for practice at home and hands-on kink workshops. This guide offers a lot of useful information to get you started, but to be a master of your craft, this is only a first step. You'll need to invest time and patience in your kink(s) of choice to perfect your skills. But, with that being said, this is a really amazing foundational step on your journey. Let's do it!

## IT CAN BE SCARY TO HAVE VULNERABLE CONVERSATIONS

First things first, talking about sex, STIs, and what we need and want can be scary. If you find going into these conversations intimidating, you are not alone. "Our sexual history is hard to talk about because most of [us] were taught by our families, culture, and religion not to talk about it," Dr. Holly Richmond, a licensed marriage and family therapist, told me in an interview. We become empowered after we choose to reject these lessons of shame and impropriety, and step into ourselves as sexually liberated people.

Now, don't get me wrong here. Getting over those internalized lessons is not easy. It takes a ton of internal growth and self-love.

Richmond says:

> When we come to a place where we understand that our sexual health is as important as our physical and mental health, we hopefully feel empowered to speak up about what we want and need, and it's mainly through trial and error in the past that we get those crucially important insights.

Through that self-growth, we have to learn an entirely new vocabulary to discuss sex. When I asked Kristine D'Angelo, a certified sex coach and clinical sexologist, about this, she said that "it's very common to feel nervous about a subject that many of us aren't used to expressing, especially verbally and to somebody we're starting to develop feelings for."

Bottom line, when you're coming into your own and embracing yourself as the sexual, fabulous, kinky B that you are, talking about sex can still be scary. Being nervous about sex and being sexually empowered are not independent of one another. They can coexist inside the extremely complex human psyche, and that is perfectly OK. Accepting this is all a part of developing self-love.

## STI PREVENTION AND SCREENING

Here is the good word: STIs are not *bad* things that only dirty people get; they're a fact of human life just like every other kind of infection for which we have methods of protection, prevention, and treatment.

STIs are incredibly common. There were more than 1.6 million cases of chlamydia reported in 2023 in the United States. One in six people currently has genital herpes. The point is, STIs happen. This is just a fact of life.

We have so much shame around STIs that we can't even understand the fact that most of them are common, easily treated, and not the end of the world. Chlamydia is easier to treat than strep throat. You take one dose of an antibiotic (yes, one single dose) and the infection is gone. Think about this for a second: When you get strep throat, you take a seven- to ten-day cycle of antibiotics to treat the infection. When you get chlamydia, you take one pill to treat the infection. And yet when you get strep, no one thinks you're a nasty, diseased person. They simply think you're a person who has a common infection and is seeking treatment. The only reason chlamydia is seen as something scarier than strep is because we're so scared of sex and place so much shame on STIs.

Taking STIs seriously doesn't require making people feel like they're a pile of human garbage for contracting one. Taking STIs seriously means presenting the facts as facts, not as an indictment of character. We need to end the stigma and take it out with the trash. Stigma doesn't prevent people from getting STIs; information does.

With that being said, practicing safer sex is crucial to keep you and your partner(s) as safe as possible. STIs are common and a part of life, but avoiding them is still a good thing.

Not all kink involves sexual touch, but that doesn't mean we shouldn't be prepared regardless. If you know you and your play partner are not going to be engaging in any sort of play that could spread STIs, OK. But if there is even a chance there could be a risk, you should always be cautious. "Knowing each participant's STI status helps mitigate the risk of transmission and ensures safer play. Discussing STI status is essential for informed consent, which is a cornerstone principle in kink activities," says board-certified sex educator Linnea Marie. "It allows everyone involved to make informed decisions about engaging in specific activities based on their risk tolerance and health concerns."

### Get tested regularly

The US Centers for Disease Control and Prevention (CDC) recommends getting tested for STIs at least once per year. If you're having regular sex with multiple partners, it's beneficial to get tested much more often. Preferably every 8–12 weeks. I always suggest getting tested after every new sexual partner.

### Talking to partner(s) about STI screening

While talking about STIs is a scary thing sometimes, we need to do it to practice safely. "Regular testing and discussions of STI status are key for exploring ethically, and encouraging individuals to take responsibility for their health," Marie says. "Discussing STI status fosters trust and communication between partners. It creates an environment where individuals feel comfortable being open, and addressing sensitive topics related to sexual health and boundaries." In kink, we're exploring quite vulnerable states of mind and body—we need to have trust with our partners to practice safely. If you don't feel safe enough to openly discuss STI status with a kink partner, it's highly unlikely you'll feel safe enough with them to play in the world of the taboo, you know?

Three tips for talking to a partner about your STI status:

I.  **Context:** You want to have discussions about STIs before any play takes place. This means considering the timing and the location of this chat. "Discussing the topic in a private, relaxed setting where all parties feel safe and feel comfortable should be prioritized," Marie says. This can easily be done over text, too. Something as simple as: "I'm really looking forward to playing together! Could you let me know when you were last tested for STIs? I'd appreciate seeing your results, as well. Happy to share mine, too."

2. **Help your partner feel safe:** Let your partner know that you prioritize sexual health and safety, and are in no way judgmental about STIs. Make sure they know that safety is a priority for you in your kink journey. "This can also help ease any potential discomfort your partner(s) may have about sharing their status, sexual history, or trauma," Marie says.

3. **Listen to the response:** If someone is a dickhead about sharing their STI status, take that as valuable information. You learn a lot about a person by how they respond to a boundary that you set. If they won't share with you or get defensive, it's likely this person is not a safe partner for kink.

### Use barrier methods

I am not even joking a little bit here: *Use condoms*. I repeat: *Use condoms!!*

Barrier methods are essential in preventing STIs. I'm talking condoms, dental dams, and gloves. "This is especially important during activities involving bodily fluids or mucous membranes," Marie says.

Keep in mind that the following STIs are not reliably prevented with barrier methods, as they are (or can be) passed skin-to-skin:

- herpes (HSV1 and HSV2)

- HPV (human papillomavirus)

- syphilis.

## STI-prevention medications and vaccines

In addition to barriers, taking STI-prevention meds is a must. Knowing about and taking preventive medications such as PrEP, Doxy PEP, and Lenacapavir can be life-changing, allowing for more pleasure and less fear. Unfortunately, Doxy PEP is still being investigated and isn't available everywhere in the world, just yet. Lenacapavir (which is used to treat HIV and AIDS) isn't available as PrEP in the UK currently, so it's always worth checking with your medical provider to see what options are available to you. It is, however, widely available in the US.

There is an HPV vaccine available to adults in most countries up to 45 years of age. This vaccine has been shown to greatly reduce HPV-causing cancers such as cervical, oral, and throat cancers. If you haven't had the vaccine, you should consider getting it!

## Clean your tools and toys

Always thoroughly clean your toys, tools, and implements between uses. When in doubt, read the instructions. This is how we prevent spreading STIs and damaging our (often quite expensive) kink equipment.

Choosing gentle products is especially important for people who have vulvas. If you own a vulva, never use soap. Soap disrupts the pH in that delicate biome and kills the good bacteria in the vagina, which can lead to microbial growth. This can lead to yeast infections, bacterial vaginosis (BV), or vaginitis. In the same vein, the vagina cleans itself (like a self-cleaning oven!) and also has a sensitive ecosystem of good bacteria. When this ecosystem is disturbed, it can wreak havoc on the vaginal biome. All you need for a happy vulva and vagina is some warm water.

No matter what kind of genitals you own, make sure that any cleanser you're buying is gentle and unscented. When in doubt, a classic Dove Beauty Bar is a solid choice.

## THE RULES OF RACK

RACK stands for "risk awareness consensual kink." This means being fully aware of what kind of play is going to take place, knowing how to do it safely, and ensuring everyone enthusiastic-ally consents. A big part of kink under the RACK framework is negotiating scenes that feel safe and pleasurable for both part-ners. While our discussion of RACK in this chapter points to elements of physical safety, the emotional side of RACK is just as important. We'll be discussing this in the next chapter. There are other consent models (such as PRICK, SSC) which you may want to research yourself outside of this book. As a therapist and kinkster, I find the RACK model to be the most effective and easy to understand, especially for beginners—so we're going to keep it nice and straightforward here with an easy-to-follow model.

In kink, no stone is left unturned. Partners take great care in discussing the finer details of a scene to ensure everyone is on the same page with the play. This is not a "go on and see what happens and then deal with the consequences later" kind of thing.

BDSM and kink play can be quite complex and risky, which means every scene needs to be highly negotiated and talked through with partners. "You need to know your own boundaries and respect your partner's boundaries, keeping in mind that the most limiting boundary is THE boundary because everyone participating needs to be safe," Criss says. This means that we need to be aware of every single boundary and work within its confines for the duration of play. No play is 100 percent safe, but by following the RACK, we can make play as safe as possible.

Remember, you are new to this, and it is going to take some practice. It's OK to acknowledge that these conversations can be super awkward. After all, it's not like any of us were ever taught how to talk about sex, let alone kink. Being willing to be vulnerable and honest within the RACK framework is a great first step.

Let's take some examples that we've already covered: age play (think: Daddy/little girl and Caregiver/little) and bondage.

### Using RACK in age play

- Do your research to ensure you know what you're doing.

- Consider exactly what both partners want out of their roles, including the names they would or would not like to be called— for example, sweetie, honey, good girl, etc.

- Lay out the outfits you envision wearing.

- Get clear on the activities you'd like to engage with, such as coloring books, spankings, or time-outs.

- Discuss safe words or safe gestures.

- If there are activities on the table that involve more skill (such as impact play or bondage), figure out if both of you have the skills to safely engage.

• Obtain and regularly check in to ensure everyone is giving enthusiastic consent throughout play.

## Using RACK in bondage

• Do your research to ensure you know what you're doing.

• Get clear on each partner's roles, how you want to be treated, and what a scene would ideally look like for you. Negotiate, negotiate, negotiate.

• Ensure lines of communication can remain open throughout the play.

• Get clear on what kinds of bondage you have on the table (examples: ropes, handcuffs, hoods, cages).

• Discuss safe words or safe gestures.

• If there are activities on the table that involve more skill (such as using ropes for tying), figure out if both of you have the skills to safely engage.

• Have necessary safety gear nearby, such as safety scissors to cut rope, if needed.

Other items you should always have nearby include:

• First aid kit with gauze, medical tape, sterile wipes, antiseptic solution, and bandages and Band-Aids for cuts and bruises.

- Lube, especially if play involves any sort of penetration. Choose something paraben and glycerine-free.

- Ice packs for any bruises or sore spots (especially after impact play).

- A sharps container to dispose of any needles (if you're practicing blood play or any play involving needs or cutting of any kind).

## VETTING POTENTIAL KINK PARTNERS

Doing your due diligence if you're playing with someone new is also important. "It's highly encouraged that [you] spend extra attention on vetting potential play partners," professional Dom, Mistress Kye, told me in an interview.

What this might look like:

- Meeting in a public place to discuss and negotiate the details of the scene and your boundaries.

- Asking for references from other people they've played with. Yes, you can really do this!

- Enquiring about the person's past experiences playing with this specific kink/type of play/scene.

The vetting of partners ensures that you're only playing with people who know what they're doing, can be trusted, and have your best interests at heart. Again, we can never be 100 percent in control over other people, but we can do due diligence to ensure we're as safe as possible.

## FIND YOUR PEOPLE

Learning about kink can also include finding a community. You can go online and search around to find your local kink community. You can choose to attend a "Munch," which is a casual gathering of kinksters to talk and get to know one another. "BDSM practitioners tend to be into education and community. If there is a group near you, they're probably hosting play parties, workshops, and mentoring newcomers," Criss says.

Finding like-minded people can make BDSM a lot more accessible and fun. Check out apps like FetLife and Feeld for Munch gatherings—or even just give it a Google search along with where you live to see if anything pops up.

## LEARNING YOUR STUFF AND PRACTICING YOUR CRAFT

To play with kink within the RACK framework, you have to learn your stuff. We're all beginners here, and it's OK to be nervous. Becoming "good" at kink takes time and patience as we nurture our skills.

This guide isn't meant to be your sole source of learning material in skills practice—and it isn't meant to give you all the information you need to learn every single kink skill there is, but it is a first resource.

Criss says you really do need hands-on training to hone your skills—and I couldn't agree more. "Curious about Shibari and suspension bondage? Take a class! If you're interested in Florentine flogging, find someone who does this and ask them to show you how," she says. "Learn about the body: Anatomy, physiology, and first aid are essential to make sure you don't hurt your partner." You need a skillful practitioner to avoid injuries, including to nerves.

For all kink play, start slowly. When it comes to gear, less is more. "A lot of people start with blindfolds, light bondage, or a little bit of spanking," Criss says. "Don't dive into the deep end with breath play/choking—that needs some skill and training to do safely." This means that since you're a fresh kinkster, the journey will mean starting with simpler stuff while you learn more complex skills. And some people may choose to stay permanently with the skill-light kink play (such as blindfolds, pegging, and certain forms of role-play)—and that is completely OK, too. You don't have to become a master kink practitioner to engage with many of the forms of kink play. It's all about what works for you and what piques your interest.

Let's break down a few examples of where skills learning needs to be prioritized to stay safe. For more resources, including classes where you can hone your skills with practitioners you can trust, check out the "resources" pages at the back of the book.*

These examples were specifically chosen to demonstrate just how many skills you need to engage with certain kinds of high-risk play safely. These examples are certainly not exhaustive, and each kink has its own skillset.

## SHIBARI

As we covered in Chapter 2, Shibari is the art of Japanese rope bondage. This form of bondage is a varsity-level form of rope tying. It takes a lot of work and training to be good at it.

Shibari instructor Julieta Chiara says that it is advised that you are fully trained as a rigger before doing Shibari—this stuff can be

---

\* For information on how to do breath play and choking, check out the next chapter where we break this down in detail.

*dangerous*. This isn't your old "throw on some handcuffs and mess around" kind of kink. It's truly a cultivated skill set.

Here are some skills to hone before trying Shibari:

◆ Start with a basic "single-column tie" (like a Somerville Bow-line). This type of tie is the first skill Shibari practitioners usu-ally learn. There are plenty of instructional videos on YouTube. Just make sure the videos you're watching are made by actual kink professionals. There is value in reading the descriptions!

◆ Start with a floor tie rather than going straight into suspension, as in, stay on the ground, don't try to use suspension hooks to dangle a partner. You want to perfect your tying abilities before taking things to the level of suspension, as this requires more skill and comes with additional safety risks.

◆ Always keep a pair of safety scissors within reach to cut the rope, if needed. If your partner is feeling uncomfortable, numb, or in pain, the rope should be cut immediately.

◆ Make sure you're playing in a safe, comfortable space where you have access to all the tools you need.

◆ Be sure you're buying the right stuff. Most practitioners suggest rope made of jute because it's a strong natural fiber. You can also opt for hemp, silk, or fiber rope.

It really is in your best interest to take in-depth classes on Shibari before giving it a go on your own or with a partner. Chiara teaches a comprehensive beginners and intermediate ropes course, which you can take in person, via Zoom, or replay at your own pace. Check out her website at www.julietachiara.com/store for more.

## IMPACT PLAY

Let's talk about one of the most recognizable forms of kink: impact play. Simply put, impact play is spanking with tools. It involves hitting or being hit using hands, paddles, floggers, canes, crops, and more. But don't be fooled by how simple it sounds—when done consciously and consensually, impact play is an art form.

Within the BDSM world, impact play allows a Dominant and submissive to explore a powerful combination of tactile sensation, pain play, physical endurance, and—let's be honest—pleasure. When done safely and intentionally, it can feel really, really good.

Here are some examples of impact play:

+ flogging

+ paddling

+ caning

+ spanking (with hands or tools)

+ using a crop.

Impact play is about more than just swinging a paddle. Here are some basics to keep in mind before getting started:

+ Learn your tools. Understand how your chosen implement works and how to use it safely. A flogger hits differently than a crop or cane. YouTube is full of demos from professional Doms—watching how they handle tools can be super helpful.

+ Pacing is key. "Go slow when you're starting out," says Criss. "Try one or two things for a short time and debrief after—what worked, what didn't, and what you'd like more of." Impact play is a shared journey, not a race.

- Start with hands first! Chiara recommends beginning with light spanking using a flat hand on the outer middle quadrant of the glutes. Play with intensity and discover what feels good for both of you before introducing any tools.

- Don't start with the heavy hitters. Avoid jumping straight into intense implements like canes. Stick with beginner-friendly options like large paddles, riding crops, or soft floggers as you build your confidence and skill.

- Know your anatomy. The safest places for impact are the buttocks and the upper thighs—these are meaty areas that can absorb sensation well. Stay away from the lower back (kidneys = vulnerable) and be mindful when experimenting with impact on areas like arms or breasts. Rule of thumb: Aim for the squishy bits.

- Remember to communicate. Impact play is intimate, and checking in throughout the scene is essential. Make sure sensations are feeling good and boundaries are being respected in real-time.

- Know basic first aid. Bruises and marks are sometimes part of the deal, so learn how to treat them safely—cold compresses and rest can go a long way.

- Practice, practice, practice. Mastery takes time. The more you practice (with intention and communication), the more confident and connected your play will feel.

Unlike rope bondage or Shibari, you don't necessarily need a full course to try impact play—but you do need communication, a basic understanding of anatomy, and a willingness to go slow and learn.

Always have a safe word ready, keep consent at the center, and remember there's no award for being the edgiest player in the dungeon—especially when you're just starting out. "There are no prizes for being the kinkiest or toughest player in the dungeon, especially if you're just starting out," Criss says.

Impact play is a skill. Take your time, build your knowledge, and, most importantly, enjoy the journey. Rushing in increases the risk of injury, which can take all the fun out of what should be a deeply connective and satisfying experience.

## BLOOD PLAY

In Chapter 4, we broke down why people are so aroused by blood in their kink play in the section on niche play. But how do you safely engage with this kink?

Coming as a surprise to no one, blood play can be quite risky. Cutting yourself or another person comes with the risk of infection or the spread of STIs. There is also the risk of scarring to consider. Former professional Dom and sex-positive therapist Ness Cooper says that the (consensual and desired) fear that accompanies bloodplay can mess with blood pressure, leading to the risk of going into shock or having a panic attack.

So, yeah, skills are needed to engage with blood play as safely as possible. Consider using fake blood first. This eliminates the risk of STI spread, scarring, and other health concerns. You should also consider other bloodborne pathogens such as Hep A, Hep C, and some parasites that appear in blood that you should be very careful of. In general, it's best to avoid drinking blood unless you're fully aware of someone's STI and health status. If you're a beginner, I highly recommend sticking with the fake stuff. It just makes everything so much easier. You can get fake blood on Amazon or at any Halloween or party store. "Blood play is not for beginners. You should already feel comfortable communicating and advocating for your sexual needs and boundaries," Sarah Melancon, Ph.D., a sociologist and clinical sexologist, told me in an interview.

Here are some skills to hone before trying blood play:

• Safety around blood play starts with everyone *wanting* to engage with it. BDSM stresses the importance of negotiation and enthusiastic consent. These same rules of consent, communication, and understanding are involved with blood play, and they are critical as blood can be dangerous (which is one reason why it can be hot).

• If you're a beginner, period sex can be a great way to engage with blood in a less dangerous way.

• Be sure you fully and clearly communicate about your STI status and any health conditions that might impact the play (such as high or low blood pressure, cardiovascular issues, and certain medications like blood thinners, etc.).

• If you decide to cut your skin or someone else's, it's crucial that you make sure the implement is fully sterilized. Be sure to have bandages and a dedicated bin specifically for any sharp objects used. After you're finished, clean any cuts with soap and water, apply an antibacterial ointment, and cover with a bandage.

• Learn proper first aid for any cuts, scratches, etc. This means having bandages, alcohol, and antiseptic ointment nearby at all times.

Learning how to do bloodplay safely really does take a lot of skill. I highly recommend learning from a qualified BDSM practitioner who has a lot of experience with blood play specifically.

## HAVE A PLAN IN PLACE IF SOMETHING GOES WRONG

Having a plan in place for if something doesn't go to plan is crucial. Sure, we don't expect things to go awry in any way, but mistakes *do* happen, and we need to prepare accordingly.

### Have safety gear ready

This means thoroughly discussing and thinking through what you would do in the case of an emergency. For example, having safety scissors nearby if you're playing with rope ensures you can quickly release a partner from ties that might be too tight.

### Pay attention to bodies and body language

Often, our bodies will tell us something is wrong before our minds have a chance to catch up. For example, if you see that someone's hands are turning slightly blue in handcuffs, or their pupils are unusually dilated during breath play, take this as a sign to pause play and check in.

This becomes easier the more you practice with kink play. You start to pick up on a lot more, which is why I, and the experts you've heard from, always emphasize taking things slowly and carefully.

### Continuously check in

Make sure check-ins are ongoing—before, during, and after play.

You want to ensure that both you and your partner are feeling safe, secure, and comfortable. Be conscious of safe words (which we'll talk more about in the next chapter). If someone calls a safe word, all play stops, and a check-in happens.

### Step out of your role

If an accident happens, you need to jump out of your D/s/Top/bottom role and into problem-solving, safety mode. The scene is halted at this point. All attention is paid to resolving the issue and taking care to make sure everyone is alright.

For even more on action plans, check out Chapter 12, which breaks down finely tuned ways to integrate kink with boundaries, consent, and accountability. In the next chapter, we'll also break down some of the mental and emotional implications of boundary crossing.

### Chapter 6 recap

In Chapter 6, we entered the Wild West of physical safety. We explored STI testing and how to approach talking to a partner about STI status. We broke down some of the stigma around STIs and even looked at a concrete example of what to say to a potential partner when you want to know when they were last tested.

Next, we broke down the RACK framework in kink. Risk-aware consensual kink is the foundational layer of ethical kink practice. Within it, we're taking care to ensure everyone is aware of the risks involved in certain kinds of play, and that everyone has the skills to safely carry out the play, and ensuring all parties are 100 percent on board and consenting to everything that happens within a scene.

This can include vetting partners to ensure the people you're playing with are safe, because, yes, you should be able to ask for references.

Next, we broke down the importance of skill enhancement and practice. Some forms of kink are more dangerous and require more expertise than others. We looked at three prime examples of this edgier play: Shibari, bondage, and blood play. Of course, there are *so* many more kinds of kink play that require special training, and I'd encourage you to research the hell out of whatever interests you.

Last, we thought through what to do if something goes wrong during a scene because accidents happen, and we need to be prepared to handle them with care.

## JOURNAL PROMPTS

1. After covering the basics of physical safety, how are you feeling about kink in your own life? Does anything stand out to you? Reflect on this.

2. What is a skill you'd like to enhance around kink? What could you do to make that happen?

3. What kind of kink play do you feel most equipped to try (e.g. role-play, light bondage, spanking, etc.)? How do you see that scene playing out? Who's in what role? Is there equipment present?

# EXERCISES

## A QUICK STI QUIZ

1.  Which three STIs cannot reliably be prevented with barrier methods?

    a.  HIV, herpes, HPV

    b.  HPV, herpes, syphilis

    c.  syphilis, HPV, chlamydia

    d.  gonorrhea, HIV, HPV

    e.  chlamydia, herpes, HPV

*Answer: b*

2.  Thinking through physical safety during a scene.

    Let's think through a scene. You're with a partner and are doing some Shibari. Assuming everyone involved in this scene has been properly trained in Shibari, what are the five things you should consider around physical safety? Consider your learning from the chapter and answer below. For additional practice, consider *why* each thing is important.

    a.                                    d.

    b.                                    e.

    c.

*Here are some possible answers:* Safety scissors, check in regularly, use safe words, pay attention to body language, use simple knots, go slowly, get consent for everything you're doing, make sure the body is responding and circulation is not cut off, and so forth.

# 7

# EMOTIONAL SAFETY

## The Basics

---

**What you'll find in this chapter:**

→ The nuances of consent in kink.

→ Consent and kink.

→ RACK.

→ Two controversial kinds of kink play that illustrate the care and education needed to engage in kink safely:

 • breath play

 • rape and ravishment fantasies, CNC play.

→ Exercises.

---

**W**e can be out here all day saying over and over again that we need to be safe when we're going to engage in kink play. We've talked about all the (rather intense, not gonna lie) rules around physical safety, but what about our sweet little emotional selves? We need to consider emotional and psychological safety with the same dedication we offer to our physical selves. Practicing kink safely means thinking about it holistically. It's not just about knowing where to keep the safety scissors during rope tying, but also checking in to make sure that your partner is feeling safe and secure during the play, both during and after. It's about obtaining ongoing, informed consent while understanding and maintaining boundaries. Now that we've considered the physical side of the RACK model, let's consider the emotional side.

The Pillars of Emotional Health and Safety:

◆  consent

◆  boundaries

◆  negotiation

◆  RACK

◆  check-ins

◆  safe words

◆  aftercare.

We'll break all of this down. Let's go!

## THE NUANCES OF CONSENT

As much as sex-positive folx love to say "Consent is sexy" and "If it isn't a 'Hell yes,' it's a 'No,'" understanding the intricacies of consent is more difficult than we might believe. It's not as simple as "Yes means yes" or "No means no" or "Maybe means no," etc.

As defined by Planned Parenthood, consent is an agreement and permission for something to happen. In relationships and sexual settings, consent should be:

- freely given
- enthusiastic
- reversible
- specific.
- informed

Carol Queen, Ph.D., the staff sexologist for feminist sex toy retailer Good Vibrations, and all-around sex ed baddie, told me in an interview that, "in a sexual context it essentially means to be *willing* to do something—and to make that clear via communication, because people have all kinds of desires, assumptions, and limits when it comes to sex."

We're all complex human beings, and consent needs to be fully and gently picked apart to fully understand it. We need to completely understand what we're saying yes to, to give informed consent. Otherwise, can we say yes to anything we experience during sex? A bit philosophical, I know, but these questions are necessary.

Since these conversations need to be handled with care, let's first start with the concept of consent more generally, and then weave those bigger themes into kink.

## THE CONFUSING STATE OF LEGAL CONSENT

Here's a rather disturbing tidbit of information you need to understand about this topic: In the US, consent—and what it means—is defined and determined on a state-by-state basis.

According to an in-depth feature by *Vice* titled "Half of the country doesn't have a legal definition of consent" (which I highly recommend reading), there is little consensus over what consent is and what it entails. As much as I'd like to throw in some elegant language to describe my feelings on this mess of a situation, all I can say is: What the actual fuck? We don't define consent federally in the US, meaning that what it means to say yes or no to a sexual act (whether that is intercourse or something else) is not recognized on a country-wide basis. Again, and I'm sure you would agree with me when I ask: What the actual fuck is going on?

There are two main ways we look at consent: "No means no," as in "if someone says no, that means no." And then there is the more recent and inclusive definition of consent: "Yes means yes." Meaning anything and everything that isn't a "yes" is a "no." Currently, California is the only state to have a "yes means yes" law on the books. I wish I were kidding, but I am not.

In the UK, things are clearer. Consent is defined as agreeing to vaginal, oral, or anal penetration by choice—and can be taken away at any time. The British understand that yes means yes, legally speaking. The law even goes so far as to say that agreeing to one sex act does not mean you are agreeing to all sex acts—a concept we'll dig into in a moment. We do love to see these more precise legal definitions. It's just mind-boggling that this isn't the way consent is defined worldwide.

## OK, LET'S DEFINE CONSENT AS BEST WE CAN

I do fully endorse the Planned Parenthood definition of consent given earlier, which says consent needs to be given freely and enthusiastically, and the consent must be specific.

What does "enthusiastic" mean? What can we take from the word "specific" in a sexual context? Queen says that enthusiastic consent is a stronger form of consent. You can feel pretty "meh" about something and still consent to it, but when it's enthusiastic, you're super excited about it. And this is important, Queen says, "because that enthusiasm might mean the person gets into the sex more, gets more aroused, may be more likely to orgasm. Lack of enthusiasm in sex isn't exactly a plus!"

Let's see if we can get a bit of clarity on what this means in a sexual context. What else can we do other than break down consent into meme-able, bite-sized chunks?

*What people often think asking for consent is*: Weird, awkward, unsexy, kills the mood, isn't revocable once given, a yes to one thing means yes to everything, a necessary but uncomfortable thing you should probably obtain before sex.

*What getting consent is*: A set of sexy questions that indicate respect for yourself and your partner, a fundamental part of good, healthy sexual experiences, revocable at any time, for any reason; a thing you *must* get before every single sex act for your actions to be ethical and legal.

*What consent also is*: Informed. Is everyone aware of what they are being offered, and do they have all the information they need to make a decision? This is so important because consent is not just about saying yes to something; it is saying yes while also knowing what is happening. You need to have all the information to truly consent to something. For example, if you want to engage in role-play, you need to be informed of the kind of role-play and the possible risks for it to be informed consent. Another example is if you have a foot fetish and don't disclose it and instead ask your partner to wear high heels during sex without any further explanation, then their consent isn't fully informed.

## The enthusiastic "maybe"

We've talked about the "enthusiastic yes" when it comes to consent. Enthusiasm is a huge part of this "yes." If enthusiasm is lacking, it's a "no." This "yes" is not a one-time conversation. It isn't a blanket affirmation that allows you to do anything you want, whenever you want.

Consent is an outline. It denotes the ways two people are going to interact with each other sexually or intimately within clearly communicated boundaries. Consent ensures that everyone involved is informed of behaviors or actions that will occur and any risks that may come with any play or behaviors, and they are enthusiastic and excited about the experience.

Enthusiasm ensures that the other person is saying "yes" because this is something they want. Enthusiastic consent is key, as each partner wants to ensure that the other is not merely consenting due to fear, guilt, etc. If it isn't a "Hell yes!" from your partner, you have to stop and check in before moving forward. Everyone deserves to feel safe and contained before doing *anything*.

This means asking how your partner is feeling. This means checking in with yourself to see if *you're* comfortable. Sex and/or kink are fun activities, but only if everyone involved is enjoying every single part of it.

Now, here is where we must hold space for nuance. As much as I'd love for it to be as simple as "Yes means yes!" and it should be "Hell yeah" or it's a "Hell no"...well, humans just aren't that super sure about everything all the time. Welcome to the *enthusiastic maybe*.

This is when you've fully discussed and negotiated trying something new but aren't sure if you're into it yet. As sex researcher and all-around sexual wellness badass Emily Nagoski has pointed out, we aren't always 100 percent on board with something we haven't actually tried. You're not going "Hell yes," but maybe you're like "Yeah! Maybe! I am down to try it!"

And that's OK! If you and your partner have openly and honestly discussed trying something and you're feeling enthusiastically *willing* to try it, that's still consent. You're open to trying it, with the caveat that you may go for it and decide, "You know what? I actually don't think this is for me." If that happens, you're more than welcome to let your partner know that it isn't working for you. Consent must always be freely given and be able to be revoked at any time, for any reason. The key to the enthusiastic maybe is that you're clearly and openly letting your partner know you're open to trying something, but it's a *maybe* on whether you'll enjoy it or want to try it again. The maybe should be at the front of the play, wherein you're continuously checking with one another to see where you are with the maybe. If something feels off, not great, or straight-up bad, stop what you're doing. This isn't a bad thing—it's how we stay safe and respect both our and our partner's autonomy.

Expecting people to always give an enthusiastic yes as the catch-all for informed consent is, frankly, reductive. It fails to capture the complexity of human sexuality and the negotiation that comes along with trying new sexual things. We need to have space for more nuanced conversations and understanding around consent so that it can be inclusive of the experiences of one and all. We need to hold space for doubt because it exists, whether we like it or not. What matters is that we're aware, stay attuned to our partners, and are intentional every step of the way.

I'll leave you with this quote from Bianca Laureano, founder of the Women of Color Sexual Health Network, in which she expresses her distaste for enshrining the enthusiastic yes as the gold standard, and instead argues for being informed about awareness and safety.

> When people say things like "enthusiastic consent," that drives me bananas. It's ableist, and people can perform enthusiasm as a safety tactic. If I say to a young person, "I know you're having a bad day, but I really need you to put on a happy face and act like you enjoy being here just for 20 minutes," my students know exactly what to do. They sit up straight. They raised their hands. They call me Miss Whatever. They know how to perform. And that's a danger, I believe.

> Because then what happens to the neurodiverse people who don't perform enthusiasm the way we expect them to? If people have in their head that enthusiastic consent does not look like how I'm behaving, then I'm not going to get what I need. It's difficult to find definitions that aren't ableist, but I define consent as: Direct words, behaviors, and actions that show a voluntary agreement to engage with others. Someone who is consenting is comfortable and aware of their surroundings and options. They are not being coerced or manipulated and are not debilitated by drugs or alcohol.

Essentially, enthusiastic consent just doesn't serve as a catch-all for the full human experience. And we need to make space for this fact and embrace nuance.

## A "yes" does not mean "yes to all"

Saying "yes" to one sexual or intimate thing does not mean you're saying "yes" to all things.

If you're wondering what that even means, you're far from alone. Most of us don't realize that when we agree to some sexual activity, we're not giving blanket consent for all sexual activity. Raise your hand if you've ever wanted to fool around, become caught up in the moment, wanted to stop midway through, and didn't think you should "cause a scene" and instead just waited for it to be over. Yeah, pretty much everyone has been there. The fact that this is a normal part of sexual experience for so many of us is disgraceful. It's a damning indictment of the way we're socialized to think about our sexual rights—or perceived lack thereof.

We need to teach sexual communication skills to everyone to ensure that no one walks away from a sexual interaction feeling violated. This means being able to discuss boundaries with a new or current partner, and ensure you're both willing, able, and open to trying a new experience before the experience happens. And we need to understand that these conversations should be ongoing because boundaries can change. Our life experiences, feelings on any given day, moods, etc., all impact whether or not we may be open to a certain sexual experience at any given time.

## THE SEXY BOUNDARIES CHECKLIST

◆ Willing and open to try a new experience.

◆ Able to try a new experience (you feel physically fit for the act in question and are sober).

- "Nos" have been considered and agreed to. (For practice, see Exercise 2 at the end of the chapter.)

- "Yeses" have been considered and agreed to. (For practice, see Exercise 3 at the end of the chapter.)

- Safe words have been established and agreed on.

It comes down to awareness. When you're informed about boundaries and what enthusiastic consent entails, and engage in play with cautious excitement, you run less of a risk of harming another person or yourself.

## HOW TO GIVE AND GET CONSENT EFFECTIVELY

You need to understand not only the definition of consent and the implications of it, but also how to both give and get it effectively. We're usually in an emotionally charged sexual or relationship interaction when we're considering consent, and that can be intense. You can never "assume" anything, Queen tells me. Every "yes" or "enthusiastic maybe" must be spoken out loud. Even if someone was into something previously, or something (such as kissing, for instance) has led to sex in the past, that doesn't mean you can assume it will this time. "You can't guess a person's sexual interests based on their gender or gender identity, their sexual orientation, or anything else—even if you've had sex with them in the past," Queen says.

It takes (at least) two people to give and receive consent. It is a give-and-take, a conversation, and it requires that you be able to effectively communicate what you want.

Pre-play consent questions:

- Can I touch you here [insert body part]?

- Do you want to do [insert sexual act]?

- Would you be open to trying [insert the thing you want to try]?

- Do you want me to [fill in the blank]?

- Can I [fill in the blank]?

- What kind of STI and pregnancy protection do you want to use?

Remember, check in periodically to ensure that consent is ongoing.

Check-in questions to try during sexual experiences:

- How are you feeling?

- Are you comfortable?

- Are you okay?

- Do you want to take a break?

- Do you like that?

- Is this OK?

- What would you like more of?

- What would you like less of?

## Accountability

Should we cross a line and impact someone's consent (i.e., if we've behaved in a non-consensual way), are we able to confront this with the person, apologize, and figure out a way to not make this mistake again?

Lucy Rowett, a certified sexologist and coach, told me in a recent interview that sex is not perfect and we sometimes make mistakes. The key is being willing to hold yourself accountable and to do what it takes to regain trust. Negotiating consent isn't always a clean-cut process. There will be misunderstandings, you will feel frustrated, and it will "go wrong" from time to time. Rowett says to think of it as a messy journey of being a human being rather than reaching the pinnacle of a "perfect" sex or kink experience.

If you cross a boundary, stop what you're doing immediately and connect with your partner. Figure out together what they need from you to rebuild trust. Humans aren't perfect, but we can become better people by acknowledging our mistakes.

## CONSENT AND KINK

### Consent and kink go hand-in-hand

Interestingly, the kink and BDSM community can teach us quite a lot about consent. As a psychotherapist who specializes in the wild world of kink, I have a deep appreciation for the kink community and its standards around consent. These folx are the ones who have it down—sustaining a long history that centers consent as a foundational principle by which play is engaged in safely. You may think that kinky people are all leather-clad daddies donning custom harnesses in the underbelly of a dungeon somewhere, mercilessly spanking the ass of a young buck in assless chaps, but this simply isn't the case. Well, yeah, sometimes leather-clad daddies smack around submissives in assless chaps, but a lot was going on behind the scenes of said assless chaps ass smacking—there was a boatload of negotiation around trust, boundaries, and, above all, consent.

Kristine D'Angelo, a certified sex coach and clinical sexologist, said in an interview that enthusiastic, ecstatic, mutual consent is what makes BDSM safe for people to explore. It establishes a container of assured respect and boundary adherence that makes this kind of play appealing to curious explorers. "The consent woven into BDSM ensures safety for those wanting to play," she says.

While the play may be inherently risky, within its framework of enthusiastic consent and skill, BDSM can be a lot safer than most run-of-the-mill sexual interactions. I'm not saying that the kink community is perfect when it comes to consent—because no one ever could be perfect—but there is a lot that can be learned, even if you're the most vanilla cutie on the planet.

As professional Dominatrix Mistress Kye puts it:

We operate in a ritual that manages all expectations from which a guideline sets the parameters of play. This lets everyone know exactly what's expected of themselves, their play partner(s), and their collective time together. These universally accepted and practiced rituals foster safe space for everyone. In safety, we can honor our boundaries and limits, our partners' boundaries and limits, our individual desires and fulfillment.

In kink, consent is fundamental. The bottom line is that some BDSM practices are quite dangerous. Think choking, bondage, spanking, etc.—we'll break down breath play/choking later in the chapter. These kinds of play are super fun and exciting, but need to be practiced with great care.

Every single aspect of BDSM play needs to be thoroughly discussed beforehand. While aspects of the play can seem "spontaneous," nothing is truly left out of a pre-play discussion. You may not know *when* your Dom is going to smack you with their paddle, but you do know they're not going to leave bruises on your bum if you've said you don't want marks.

## LIVE AND DIE BY THE RACK

We need to eat, sleep, and breathe the rules of RACK. As we covered in the previous chapter, RACK stands for risk awareness consensual kink. This means being fully aware of what kind of play is going to take place, knowing how to do it safely, and ensuring everyone enthusiastically consents.

Now, it may seem like I'm out here beating a dead horse with all this consent stuff, but RACK offers a tangible framework for the inherent physical and emotional risks involved in many forms of kink play. As Julieta Chiara, a kink instructor, writer, and sex expert, told me in an interview on BDSM and consent, it forms a foundation for communication, negotiation, and adherence to boundaries.

Risk awareness (recap):

+ Understand the play you're involved in and why.

+ Get educated about the physical and emotional safety needed for this kind of play.

+ Put a framework in place to mitigate risk for all partners.

Consensual kink:

+ All people involved are consenting adults.

+ All parts of play are negotiated.

+ Boundaries are understood and always respected.

- Consent can be revoked at any time. Each party should feel safe to revoke consent if needed.

- Safe words are in place to indicate when a boundary is (or is close to being) reached.

- Aftercare plans are put in place.

## NEGOTIATION

A big part of kink under the RACK framework is negotiating scenes that feel safe and pleasurable for both partners.

Let's pop back to the example of age play from Chapter 4. In age play, adhering to the rules of RACK might include considering exactly what both partners want out of their roles, including the names they would or would not like to be called. For instance, you may be A-OK with being called "honey," "baby girl," or "good girl," but being called "daddy's little slut" might be completely off the table. You really want to be crystal clear about what you want from the play before engaging in it.

You need to go through a scene (a fantasy acted out in real life) thoroughly with whoever you're playing with. For example, if you're playing with bondage, you need to negotiate your limits and what you're interested in trying. Your partner should do the same. It's all about creating a context where both people are safe and enjoying the experience.

Remember, you are not entitled to have your needs met by a partner. A specific kink or sex act can be a part of play if all parties involved are excited about it, or at least very open to it (aka an enthusiastic maybe, only kinkier).

## BOUNDARIES

In RACK, we're all about boundaries, boundaries, boundaries. Every single person in a kink scene deserves to have their boundaries understood and respected. As part of the negotiation process, be sure each person has a chance to lay out their specific boundaries. This could look like staying away from certain body parts, types of play, pieces of play equipment, etc.

## SAFE WORDS

Safe words and boundaries go together like condoms and lube. Kink can bring up a lot of emotions, so having a safe word in place acts as a way to halt play if unexpected or distressing things come up for you. You're always allowed to stop if something feels off, unsafe, or uncomfortable. Listen to yourself and honor your feelings.

Safe words are non-sexual words that indicate that you are reaching or have reached a boundary. If a safe word is called, all play should stop immediately. I suggest using the traffic light system if you're a beginner.

Red = Stop.

Yellow = I'm coming up to a boundary and might need to check in.

Green = Everything is great, and I'm loving this.

Using simple phrases like "Stop," and "I need a break" is totally OK—as long as your scene partner knows these are phrases you might use instead of a safe word, and if it doesn't contradict the scene setup, which may cause confusion. I've also offered a bunch of fun safe words in this book for you to choose from, if you'd prefer!

It's not just subs who get to have safe words. Tops are also entitled (and encouraged!) to have safe words. Safe words apply to everyone, in every kink situation and should always be respected. Just because someone is "leading" a scene, that doesn't mean they don't have their own boundaries or certain kinds of play they don't want to engage in.

## AFTERCARE AND CHECK-INS

And because kink is so much, it can bring up a lot of negative post-play emotions (such as shame and regret). Which is why we have aftercare—emotional safety, remember? Having a space where partners can connect, cuddle, and talk through feelings can help all parties feel positive about the play.

And check in! Don't just send your partner off into the world and not text or call. It's good practice to check in with a nice little "How are you feeling?" or "I had a great time with you. Just wanted to make sure you're feeling good about everything" text. It's called manners, henny.

And check-ins apply to people in relationships, too. It can be really useful to have a check-in once or twice a week on how both parties feel in the relationship and with the kinds of play they're partaking in. In kink dynamics (and all relational dynamics, tbh), we need to cultivate a communicative atmosphere so that everyone has an opportunity to regularly voice their needs and make adjustments where necessary. Some triggers are unknown and that is something both parties in a scene need to be aware of as a possibility. Triggers happen and we have to be mindful of this. With care and understanding that we may not know a trigger until we're faced with one, we can take time to connect and re-ground ourselves, even when something doesn't go to plan.

We'll take a deep dive into safe words and aftercare action plans later in the book. Stay tuned.

## THE KINKY CONSENT CHECKLIST

+ A clear verbal statement of "yes" (or an enthusiastic maybe—with regular check-ins) has been given.

+ Consent has been willingly and enthusiastically given by the person you want to engage with.

+ The scene has been thoroughly discussed and negotiated.

+ Boundaries are clear and understood.

+ The person(s) who is consenting is sober and unimpaired.

+ It is clearly understood that this consent is only valid for the activity for which it was originally given.

+ It is clearly understood that consent can be withdrawn at any time.

+ It is clearly understood that consent can change or be altered by both parties when communicated, at any time.

+ All parties are aware of the cultural, relational, and personal power dynamics (and imbalances) within this interaction.

+ There are safe words in place to ensure consent is ongoing and boundaries are communicated.

+ Check-ins are considered, agreed to, and ongoing.

+ An aftercare plan is in place to discuss the activities the parties have consented to.

Everyone feels safe and ready to play.

## EXAMPLES THAT ILLUSTRATE SAFETY AND CARE AROUND HIGHER-RISK PLAY

Are there any juicy examples of kink play that truly illustrate the care and education needed to engage in kink safely? Hell yeah: breath play and CNC.

Kink is very, very (very, very, very) misunderstood and often thought to be violent, dangerous, bad, and generally wrong. But this couldn't be further from the truth. Given that we've taken some glorious time to break down consent and the RACK to its nuts and bolts, you can hopefully see by now that when done with care and intentionality, kink is centered on safety, as well as all the fun, sexy stuff.

With all of this newly acquired safety information in our toolkit, let's examine two prominent examples of where kink is unfairly painted as violence: breath play and CNC. I've chosen choking and rape fantasy intentionally because they are two of the most misunderstood and demonized forms of kink play. Using what we know from the RACK, I'd like us to take a closer look at these acts because, for the anxious overthinkers among us, education is key to understanding and integration.

Trigger warning: If reading about breath play or CNC fantasies feels upsetting to you, skip to the chapter exercises and journal prompts below. Always take care of yourself first.

### Example #1: Breath play (aka choking)

Breath play may be the most controversial kink out there at the moment—if only because of its presence in the mainstream media. There are a lot of ongoing discussions around choking right now, and for good reason! Choking someone during sex is dangerous.

I need to be 100 percent clear that choking someone during sex is never actually safe. In fact, recent research has shown that any amount of choking can lead to brain damage. A lot of people may be aware that choking can lead to serious injury and death, but they may not realize that it can actually cause brain damage, regardless of how you do it. And while I could sit here and say "JUST DON'T DO IT!" I believe that is a disservice. Because people DO do this. And so, the best I can do is try to help you make this play as safe as I can. With education and care, we can aim to reduce risk as much as possible.

While choking will always come with risks and can't be done with 100 percent safety, if you and a partner choose to engage in choking during sex, you need to fully understand the risks and learn what you're doing to mitigate them as much as possible. This is my goal here.

We're seeing a rise in young people casually employing choking as a normal part of hookups. In 2020, a national survey of Americans aged 18 to 60 years found that 21 percent of cisgender women reported having experienced choking during sex. Twenty percent of men reported that they had choked a partner during sex. According to the UK-based Institute for Addressing Strangulation, within the 16–34 age group surveyed, 35 percent of respondents reported having been choked during consensual partnered sex. Seventeen percent of respondents reported having been choked without consent. This is so scary because these are uninformed people who are haphazardly choking their partners without understanding or living by RACK.

Why are people just casually choking everyone they have an opportunity to see naked? Because they see it in porn. This actually isn't porn's fault. Porn is entertainment. Porn is not sex education, but without proper sex ed in schools, it's unfortunately become the default education. Since porn is so much a part of our cultural experience, people think they can just run out and choke someone without understanding the safety concerns.

Let's be crystal clear here: Just because you saw it in porn does *not* mean you have an all-access pass to choke someone. You risk causing brain damage or death. Once again for the cheap seats in the back: *Seeing choking in porn does not mean you should choke someone or that you know how to choke someone.*

Here is the kicker: Choking is never entirely safe. No medical professional is ever going to tell you that choking can be done safely. When I spoke to professional Dominatrix Eva Oh about choking and safety, she pointed out that this is considered edge play—that is, play that plays with danger.

With that being said, choking *can* be done more safely if you know what you're doing. Choking someone *is* dangerous, but we can mitigate some of the risk with education and care. You certainly wouldn't know any of the safety stuff based on some of the hysterical media portrayals, which equate careful and intentional breath play with actually trying to harm someone.

Kink is centered on education. If we openly and honestly educated young people about the dangers of choking and gave them the information they needed to make the play as safe as possible, we'd all be a lot better off. Trying to hide the information and denying people education is harmful and can ultimately be what causes damage. Trying to withhold information in the hopes that people won't engage in the behavior is giving mad purity culture vibes. You can tell people not to engage in breath play, but they're still going to do it, only unsafely.

So, let's talk about breath play and how it is done with safety in mind. Because it *is* capital "D" dangerous. But that doesn't mean it can't be done with care.

So, first, why are people into it? Well, playing with breath increases arousal and intensifies orgasm. Eva Oh points to the restricted oxygen as a cause of excitement. It "translates to some people as a loss of control, another state of being [in the] mind, and I think that this is probably a huge thrill for people," she says. "It's a very harsh and present way of experiencing a loss of control, not only psychologically but physically and to quite [a] large effect."

There is also powerplay involved. The partner doing the choking may feel very primal or dominant, which can be a turn-on. The person being choked may enjoy the feeling of "helplessness" and submission that comes with this sort of play. Eva Oh shared that there can be a deeply shared intimacy that is formed in breath play, as it requires so much trust between partners. Choking may not seem like something that would facilitate bonding on its surface, but that doesn't mean bonding isn't a factor in its appeal.

When I asked Lia Holmgren, intimacy expert and author of *Play with Power*, what makes breath play such a draw for folx, she had this to say:

> Choking is an act of surrender, when we completely trust the other, dominant party and let them take complete "life-threatening" control over the submissive party. "Life-threatening" is of course just the imagination and fantasy—nobody really wants to put their life in danger—but the imagination of having no other choice and being in danger or on mercy of someone we are submissive to is sexually arousing for [the] submissive individual.

This turn-on has deep psychological implications that can allow us to explore different roles during sex.

Choking highlights the giving and receiving of control. Giving someone permission to choke you, or vice versa, allows us to take on dominant and submissive roles in bed. This is something many people crave: a release from control or the power to take it. Consensually, of course.

There is a fantasy of breath play being life-threatening, to be sure. But the "life-threatening" aspect of choking is a *fantasy*. You're not really looking for any sort of near-death experience, but the prospect of someone having that power can be hot.

## Six kinkster-approved rules for safe breath play

### 1. A clear mind is a must

There are many reasons why choking might be something that turns you on, but there are ways to do it right and ways to do it wrong. If you don't know what you're doing, haven't discussed boundaries, and aren't in a proper state of mind, stay the hell away from breath play of any kind.

If you are going to be choking your partner, you need to make it RACK. You need: risk awareness, education and training, and informed consent.

### 2. Consent, consent, consent

I might sound like a broken record here, but consent is a *must* when it comes to all play, especially play that involves risk. This means a clear, ongoing yes. You should regularly check in with your partner to make sure they are OK. Use your safe words liberally, where needed. Keep in mind that, as of the date of publication, strangulation is an offense in the UK and, if serious harm occurs, consent is not a defence. This means you are taking a risk by engaging in this play, even if you do it with safety in mind. You should make sure you and your partner(s) are familiar with the laws of the country you are in. I say this as a precaution. Yes, adults can engage in any play they want if everyone is enthusiastically consenting, even if it isn't legal, but the risk is there, nonetheless. You deserve to have all the information possible to make the most informed choices about what you do or do not do with a partner. Keep in mind that while this is the case in the UK, there may be different laws in other countries. I encourage you to learn about the laws of the country you are in currently and the laws in the country where you are originally from.

### 3. Take classes and learn what you're doing

If you don't know what you're doing, you could seriously hurt someone.

The way to figure out how to choke someone is with workshops, proper training, and practice. If you're seriously interested, seriously learn about it. Study anatomy and take kink classes led by respected practitioners.

This is a sex act that has serious repercussions if done incorrectly. You are restricting airflow, but that doesn't mean you should be crushing your partner's esophagus or putting your entire weight on their neck.

### 4. Pay attention

Be aware of what you're doing and how your partner responds. The bottom line is that if you restrict someone's airflow for too long, you can legitimately cause brain damage or death, so you have to stay present. Be intentional during play to ensure the safest experience for both yourself and your partner.

When we're close to orgasm, our bodies become less aware of pain. Always be cautious with choking—think of it more as breath play in general. Your partner should be able to answer you if you speak. If they can't, stop what you're doing immediately. Never choke someone so hard that they cannot express words vocally.

Check in with one another and gather information about personal preferences as you become more experienced.

### 5. Set up boundaries

Yes, we are back to boundaries! Before any choking takes place, both partners need to establish boundaries and indicate what each person is and isn't OK with.

Perhaps you're looking for "hands-only" play wherein a partner only uses their hands to choke you. Maybe a collar or rope is more your thing? Whatever it is you're into, a discussion must take place first. According to Holmgren:

> The boundaries you want to focus on when choking [are] to establish the timing or goal of choking, either as part of a fantasy or to increase the intensity, and discuss how long the choking might last. You want to determine when your partner wants to be choked (during penetration, oral, etc., or closer to climax).

Boundaries to consider:

* Establish the timing or goal of choking, as Holmgren says, either as part of a fantasy or to increase the intensity.

* Discuss how long the choking might last.

* Discuss and determine when your partner wants to be choked—is it during penetrative sex? During oral sex? When they're about to orgasm? Get clear!

### 6. *Have a safe word*

In all BDSM play, a safe word should be established beforehand. A safe word is an agreed-upon, usually non-sexual, phrase that indicates when one's partner is uncomfortable and wants the play to stop. Holmgren says that when we're talking about breath play, or any BDSM play that involves vocal restriction, a safe "signal" might work best. She suggests "tapping three times" as a good alternative to a spoken safe word.

Additionally, there is an element of the "style" in which you're using choking. Is it playful, dominant, or maybe a little scary? All of this should be determined *before* you ever choke someone.

Choking is never completely safe, OK? It is a dangerous act and anyone thinking about including choking in their play should fully educate themselves on the safety and legal risks of this kind of play.

But, like I said, people do engage in it so I always want to encourage people to learn what can be done to reduce risk as much as possible.

My position is not: "Choking is safe if you do it my way." My position is: "Choking is dangerous and never fully safe, but if you're going to do it, let me try to help you make it as safe as possible."

## Example #2: Consensual non-consent (CNC), aka rape fantasies

A second example of an often completely misunderstood kink is rape fantasy—or CNC. I think breaking down and understanding CNC does a lot to show just how careful, intentional, and planned kink play is.

Believe it or not, I receive a question in my inbox from someone wanting to try ravishment scenes at least a few times each month. I know, given the current political and social climate, discussing rape as a part of sexual fantasy may feel a bit tone-deaf. Look, I get it. But, that being said, rape fantasy is so common.

Let's talk a little about how "normal" a certain kind of fantasy may be. There is no "normal" when it comes to sexual turn-ons. If something turns you on sexually and is not harming another person in any way, it's OK to think about it. A fantasy is a game—it's a sexual illusion. The human mind is a miraculous thing, capable of imagining all sorts of wild and amazing stuff.

We live in a sexually repressive society. We're fed messages of *abstinence-only*, and "sex is bad," and "what feels good is not good for you" all the time. Because of this onslaught of *wrongness* surrounding sex, we begin to sexualize what is taboo. Sex is taboo, something we cannot have open conversations about. Therefore, we're left with our imaginations. The more society tells you you're not supposed to want or like something, the more you want it. Minds are funny that way.

Now, let's narrow in on rape fantasy, specifically. A rape fantasy is not *actual* rape. This is possibly the *most* important point here. Rape is when a person is sexually forced against their will and their consent is stripped away from them. It is a traumatic, violent, violating thing that no one should ever have to experience. Rape *fantasy*, on the other hand, is consensual, negotiated, and planned.

Rape fantasy has come to be known by the more culturally sensitive term CNC. But no matter what you call it, people do have this fantasy and often wish to pursue it. A CNC *fantasy* is a deeply communicated, well-planned, *consensual* role-play scene. It is not about being violated or put in actual harm; it's the illusion of that scenario. It's about having our control taken away from us, in a controlled way. To play out a CNC fantasy, there is no actual sexual assault taking place.

There are many reasons *why* we have these fantasies, but none of them imply that we want to be attacked or violated in a literal sense; it means we want to be "ravaged" in a negotiated setting. This means having safe words, knowing exactly when and how things are going to go down, and having regular check-ins to make sure everyone is comfortable.

Both partners need to be fully on board with the scene and give informed consent. Playing out any form of sexual role-play takes trust. Empathy is also key here. Partners need to have a thorough, honest conversation about the scene and their boundaries.

Remember, you don't have to do anything you don't want to do. You never have to engage in an act of any kind. I'll say this again and again: We aren't obligated to do anything we don't want to do—ever.

Yes, trying new things in bed is exciting, and I always love to encourage people to explore outside of the box, but if CNC is *not* something you're interested in doing, you don't have to. There should never be an instance where a person is doing something they feel uncomfortable with to please their partner. That isn't good sex— that's coercive. You're not going to gain pleasure from that experience, something both partners have a right to strive for. This needs to be something you both want to try for it to be positive.

Start small. Always openly communicate about what is or isn't working for you. Remember, kink has to follow the rules of RACK to be done ethically.

And when it comes to what people might *think* about your fantasies and role-play, well, what happens between consenting adults is no one else's business.

OK, we've made it to the end of a meaty chapter. How are we doing, kink-curious folx? Hanging in there? Congratulations! You've learned the basics of safety in kink play. You're one step further on your kinky journey! I'm very proud of you.

## Chapter 7 recap

In Chapter 7, we got hot and heavy with the rules for emotional safety in kink. We started with the nuances of consent, then moved on to the application of consent in kink play and how to be sure everyone is feeling safe, seen, and heard. We finished up by applying the rules of RACK to our emotional well-being when playing with darker themes or edgier play.

Last, we explored two of the most controversial kinds of kink play: breath play and CNC. These two forms of play hone in on the need for solid education and risk awareness, because they can be physically and emotionally dangerous. It doesn't mean you can't engage in these kinds of play; you just have to know what you're doing.

Taking care of your emotional well-being is critical when we're playing with kink. But with this chapter under your belt, you can hopefully start to feel more confident in your practice.

## EXERCISE 1: Identifying triggers

Think of a time in the past when you've felt suddenly frightened during an otherwise "normal" experience. This can be an intimate or sexual experience, but it doesn't have to be. Consider an experience that was not harmful or traumatic, but may have made you feel uneasy for reasons you're unsure of.

Why are we doing this uncomfortable thing? Beginning to pick apart events that left us feeling frightened or unsettled can help us identify triggers. Keep in mind that some triggers are unknown to us—and may only be identified during or after play. When we keep this in mind, we can prepare ourselves for this reality. If this happens to you, remember to take time to self-sooth, communicate with your partner (if you're with a partner), and be gentle with yourself.

*Note:* This should not be an instance of sexual assault or violation.

Write down three things that are happening in your body as you consider this event.

1.

2.

3.

Write down three things that were happening in the environment at the time. What stands out to you?

1.

2.

3.

Write down three things you remember about the person or people who were present at the time.

1.

2.

3.

Write down three emotions or feelings that are coming up for you right now.

1.

2.

3.

Write down three thoughts that are coming up for you as you do this exercise.

1.

2.

3.

Take some time to reflect on anything that jumps out at you from your lists. Does anything on your lists feel like a possible trigger? Does a specific moment come to mind? What did you do to feel calm or less panicked in this situation?

Please keep your emotional safety in mind. If thinking about these past events is upsetting, stop and take care of yourself. Take a few deep breaths and go do something that feels grounding for you.

Some grounding ideas:

- Bake something you love.
- Take a bath.
- Read your favorite book.
- Turn on your favorite playlist and dance it out.
- Call a friend and catch up.

- Pet your dog or cat.
- Scream into a pillow.
- Go get some exercise.

**EXERCISE 2:** Think about consent

Jacob and Michael are planning to engage in a spanking scene. Jacob is the Dom, and Michael is the sub. They plan to use ropes to tie Michael's hands to the bed before the scene. What needs to happen for Michael and Jacob to both fully give consent? (Hint: Think about consent and RACK.)

**EXERCISE 3:** Boundaries and defining your "nos"

Consider your go-to kinky fantasy. It can be helpful to reflect on your favorite erotic material or a fantasy scenario you use during solo sex.

Example: You're tied up like a human chandelier in a Shibari rope masterpiece. Your partner is using all kinds of toys and tools on you. The scene had been negotiated and fully consented to before play began. RACK is front and center.

Feel free to use the example above if you're having trouble visualizing your own scene.

Write down five boundaries you'd want to tell your scene partner.

(Examples: no spanking, no using the word "bitch," no using nipple clamps, no slapping in the face, no marks.)

1.

2.

3.

4.

5.

**EXERCISE 4**: Boundaries and defining your "yeses"

Now that you've defined some "nos," take some time to define some "yeses" using your imagination or the example from Exercise 3.

Write down five yeses you'd want your scene partner to be aware of during this scene.

(Examples: call me a good girl, spank my bum, use handcuffs, use vibrators.)

1.

2.

3.

4.

5.

## JOURNAL PROMPTS

1. Think back to a time when you had a truly amazing sexual experience. What made that experience so great? Try to reflect beyond the sex acts themselves and look deeper at the overall themes, using the tenets of RACK to guide you.

2. Think of a time when you felt safe during a sexual experience, solo or partnered. What about that experience made you feel safe? (Examples: your partner, the environment, the communication, the kind of sex you were having)

3. Now is your time to get creative. Take a few minutes to write out a secret fantasy that centers on consent as a main theme.

# 8

# KINK AS THERAPY

## How Some Folx Use Kink for Healing

**What you'll find in this chapter:**

→ Debunking myths about BDSM being related to mental illness.

→ How kink and BDSM can be used as tools for healing trauma.

S ince we've taken a look at some of the basics of kink safety—both physical and emotional—let's take an opportunity to dive deeper into the mental health benefits of kink. Kink is not therapy, and it isn't a replacement for therapy, but that doesn't mean it can't have therapeutic elements for people who engage in it.

As we covered earlier in the book, it's a common (and deeply messed-up) misconception that people who like kink are suffering from mental illness or some form of deep trauma. This is simply sex-negative nonsense fed to us by our puritanical culture. All kink is completely fine and normal, as long as everyone involved is a consenting adult.

We're very here for autonomy, folx. Frankly, it's not anyone's business what happens sexually between consenting adults, so this intense obsession with trying to police other people's behavior is tired as all hell—and borderline creepy if you ask me.

The misconceptions surrounding kink are mostly related to BDSM play, rather than all kink play. This is likely because in BDSM we're often playing with varying degrees of pain play, bondage, and other things that get the "average viewer's" panties in a twist.

So, for illustration, we're going to use BDSM as an example here, because that's the kind of play that most people associate with kink, in large part because of the success of *Fifty Shades*. You'll see me use kink and BDSM somewhat interchangeably throughout the next section, which many people (even seasoned kinksters) often do, but as we've established, BDSM is a form of kink play under a larger umbrella.

Studies have shown that people who engage in kink are not mentally ill—science, babies! A recent 2020 study published in the *Sexuality Research and Social Policy* shows that people who participate in BDSM score nearly the same on all relevant measures of psychological health as the general population, have similar levels of trauma and childhood experience, and have similar levels of relationship health. The skinny on BDSM is that most people who are exploring this play are doing so because it's incredibly fun and sexy, and a tool for self-actualization.

Now, this is where it gets interesting. Kinksters aren't automatically dealing with mental health problems or trauma, but some of them might be! Taylor Sparks, an intimacy educator and founder of the BIPOC-owned sex toy retailer OrganicLoven, shared with me that while mental health issues aren't usually the entry point for most, that doesn't mean they *can't* be. All humans have their shit, after all. And just because something isn't therapy, doesn't mean it can't have therapeutic benefits.

While it is most certainly true that people engage with kink because it's fun, some people utilize the unique power dynamics, pain play, and role-play involved in kink to process their personal trauma. For those who use it in this way, it can be deeply healing.

I cannot stress enough that BDSM does not nullify the importance of traditional talk therapy. Therapy is incredibly beneficial for processing trauma. But it isn't the only tool. BDSM can be used as another tool in the old belt to help people cope with the pain of their pasts. There is no right way to heal. There is only the right way for *you* to heal.

I always suggest being in therapy before engaging with kink as an outright trauma-healing tool. Using BDSM can be liberating for some people struggling with trauma or mental illness, but it also has the potential to be triggering. This is something both you and a qualified therapist should discuss before you begin engaging in kink.

In that same vein, you may be using kink already and are unaware of *why* exactly you're drawn to it. This is something to consider and reflect on to help you on your journey of self-discovery.

With all that being said, therapy can be highly restrictive due to cost, so it may not be possible for everyone to combine their kink play with outside therapy, and that's OK. There is no right or wrong way to heal, as long as we stay aware. If we're being intentional with our play and considering *why* we're drawn to it—while staying curious and conscious of possible triggers—it has the potential to be beneficial for our well-being.

Let's take a closer look at BDSM and how some folx may use it for healing.

## BDSM'S EMPHASIS ON BOUNDARIES AND CONSENT CREATES A SAFE CONTAINER

The BDSM and kink community is grounded in consent. After experiencing trauma or mental health challenges, BDSM and kink can provide a container of safety that makes it possible to explore in a way that feels approachable. "The thing I love about the kink community is the amount of education around sexuality, communication, and consent that goes along with it," says sex therapist Moushumi Ghose (who you might remember from Chapter 3's exploration of fetish). Kinksters don't just jump into scenes willy-nilly. They dutifully and cautiously discuss and negotiate every aspect of the scene to ensure everyone is playing in a way that feels good for them. This is such a severe departure from what a wounded person may have experienced in sex (and life) in the past that it can help to rebuild their sense of autonomy. Groundedness is essential for healing, and being able to explore different sensations, desires, and fantasies with partners who respect your limits and show you they care is deeply healing. It's this first layer of consent that allows people healing from trauma to begin to engage with those wounds in the context of kink.

## HOW BDSM CAN HELP SOMEONE WHO
## HAS BEEN THROUGH A TRAUMA

Working through a past trauma can be a happy byproduct of one's BDSM practice. When we experience trauma, whatever that trauma may be, and we don't process it, it lives in our bodies. As Bessel van der Kolk, MD, explains in his book, *The Body Keeps the Score*, traumas live inside of us, festering, infiltrating many areas of our lives before we properly work through them in order to heal. In many instances of macro-trauma—that is, major traumatic events—we often feel that our sense of control has been taken from us, and we disconnect from our bodies. The damage done to the nervous system results in a perpetual state of fight or flight, the body's natural response to danger. It makes healing and moving forward very difficult without professional assistance in the form of trauma-informed therapy.

BDSM can allow trauma survivors, and sexual assault survivors specifically, to regain some of the control that was robbed from them. For those in the submissive role, BDSM can be a way for them to take back control, as they are in the driver's seat of everything that is happening to them. Being submissive is a way to release residual fear and anxiety by being willing to give control to their dominant partner in a safe and controlled environment. The good old container of safety that comes from following RACK. As Ghose puts it:

Most trauma is done to us, most people who experience trauma are victims. In a kink setting, we are in control. We get to say what happens, when it happens, we get to experience pain and pleasure when we say it's OK, and with the cooperation of a (play) partner who respects us, hears us, supports us. This is the definition of loving. And, this is the opposite of trauma. We get to experience the same type of things we experienced in our trauma, but in a way that empowers us, emboldens us, and lets us take the reins. This provides us with a *corrective emotional experience* which is healing.

In BDSM, scenes are highly negotiated between sub/Dom partners to ensure complete, ongoing consent and adherence to boundaries. This gives the players the ability to create any scene they choose. This may even consist of creating scenes where the trauma is recreated. For some, reenacting their assault can help allow them to rewrite their own stories from a place of agency. Essentially, they reframe the narrative from victim to person of agency.

For others, it may be less about recreating the scene itself and more about manifesting an environment where they can release the trauma held in their bodies. The use of pain play, impact toys, restraints, and other BDSM tools can allow a person healing from trauma and an outlet for some of their pain. The physical pain helps to move the emotional pain out of the body. For some, this can be extremely cathartic.

For others still, they may engage in consensual voyeurism or exhibitionism as a way to take back control of their sexuality, watching sex acts or being watched, without fear of violation. One of the beautiful things about BDSM is its diversity. There are so many opportunities to explore every fantasy you've ever had in one space. This makes it easily adaptable to the needs of each person's healing journey. It's an opportunity to let go of shame, heal, and accept yourself.

The research on how kink can aid in healing trauma is still developing, but there have been some studies that show that engaging in BDSM can help submissive partners access altered states of awareness. This is commonly called "subspace," and is akin to a meditative relaxation state. This can offer a great sense of relief to those who are struggling with mental health issues or trauma, as they're offered a respite from suffering and have an opportunity to feel relaxed, held, and safe. They can let go and feel assured that they will be looked after by their Dom. Having that sense of safety restored is powerful.

Additionally, practicing kink with a partner can improve communication and boundary setting, which all help to solidify agency after a traumatic experience. This play can legitimately help you learn to speak up for yourself with confidence, with partners who will welcome it.

For trauma survivors, feeling at home in your body and safe with the people you're spending time with is a beautiful step toward healing. While therapy is great, if BDSM aids a trauma survivor in this way, that's fantastic. We should celebrate every fruitful healing journey, no matter how unorthodox.

## HOW BDSM AND KINK CAN IMPROVE OVERALL MENTAL WELLNESS

BDSM is, of course, not just for trauma healing. It is accessible to anyone and everyone who wants to play. For those who practice, BDSM helps foster a sense of overall well-being. It can help with improved confidence, the release of sexual shame, community building, and greater self-esteem.

When we engage in kink that feels safe, exciting, and authentic for us, we benefit from the release of feel-good endorphins and a decrease in the stress hormone cortisol. A good "scene" that is negotiated and done with care can be beneficial in your relationship with your partner as you build trust, knowing that your dominant partner always has your best interests in mind. Engaging in kink improves communication skills, as both the Dominant and the submissive learn to "use their words" to be open and honest about their kink(s), boundaries, and needs.

As Sparks puts it:

> For those who are submissives it is a way for them to take control of the outcome of what is happening to them. It is a way to release fear and anxiety by giving up the control to their dom/domme and know that they are in a safe and controlled environment. For those that are dominant it can be similar in the opposite way. This is a way to control with consent and not to worry that their urge to spank or tie someone up is "not normal."

Kink can be liberating, joyful, and healing in so many ways. It's not about being extreme and enduring; it's about finding yourself and exploring in ways that are fun and freeing.

### Chapter 8 recap

Chapter 8 is where we fully debunk the idea that people who enjoy kink and BDSM are somehow troubled, unwell, or deeply traumatized. There is so much shame-based nonsense out there about kink and the people who enjoy it. These beliefs only cause harm and make people feel alone. In Chapter 8, we tried to unravel these falsehoods and embrace our desires.

Last, we looked at how kink can help us heal from trauma and improve overall mental well-being. Some people do use BDSM and kink to help heal from trauma, and that is OK. Kink can be incredibly healing. If we practice with intention and care, we're doing it right.

## JOURNAL PROMPTS

1. Do you remember a time when you felt happy or euphoric after sex, whether kinky or vanilla? Reflect on that experience. Consider what it was about this experience that made it feel so significant. If this isn't something you've experienced before, reflect on what it might be like to have an experience like this—use your imagination!

2. After reading this chapter, breaking down the therapeutic benefits of kink, reflect on how you're feeling and what might be coming up for you. Do these ideas resonate? Does the content feel familiar? Does it feel uncomfortable or prickly in some way? Take some time to journal.

# PART III

# INTEGRATION

### Exploring Your Authentic Kinky Self

# 9

# GETTING TO THE BOTTOM OF YOUR KINKS AND TAPPING INTO THE EROTIC MIND

**What you'll find in this chapter:**

➔ What are you into?

➔ Understanding the erotic mind.

➔ How to discover what you're into when it comes to kink: Yes, No, Maybe lists and erotic content using journaling.

➔ Agony Aunt questions and answers.

➔ Exercises: Yes, No, Maybe list, mapping the erotic mind, and grounding exercises for anxious folx to try before you play.

**W**elcome to Part III! Can you believe we've made it this far? By now, you should feel pretty versed in how kink works and where it comes from, and knowledgeable in the basics of how to get started in a safe and intentional way. With all of this valuable information under your belt, you're now ready to shift your sights inward toward your kinks—to unpick what it is you like and want, and how to start integrating these likes and wants into your real-life sex life.

## HOW TO FIGURE OUT WHAT YOU'RE INTO

For many of us, getting kinky sounds very exciting. The idea of being tied up (or tying someone up) and spanking them into oblivion while wearing a leather corset and thigh-high boots is enticing—but we're just not even sure where to begin with such a fantasy because we have no idea if we're actually into something or just like the idea of it. This disconnect can be further aggravated by feelings of shame and a lack of solid educational materials available for the kink-curious among us.

Further still, you might not even have fully formed fantasies or desires quite yet. It is possible (and normal) to have vague inklings of wanting to be submissive and degraded, etc., but not be entirely sure how that would look for you. Or maybe you want to step into your power as a Dom who enjoys doling out spankings and punishments, but you're scared shitless because you don't know what kind of Dom you'd even be or even how to Dom in the first place. And what kind of implements would you even want to use, anyway?

Honestly, a lot of kink educational materials that are available kind of miss this piece of the puzzle: How do you figure out what you're even into?

Now, you might be 100 percent sure what kinds of kink play

you're into and what you want to try—and that's simply fantastic. But I would still invite you to look a bit deeper with conscious curiosity to:

1.  figure out if there are *more* kinks you're into that you're just not aware of yet

2.  understand what it is about your kinks that gets you going so intensely

3.  consider how might want to explore these kinks in your own erotic life.

Another pivotal question worth pondering: How important are these kinks to you? You might not have the answer right now—and that's OK!—but if you're here reading this book, you might have very strong kinky predilections. The first place to start is a little self-reflection.

Things to ask yourself:

◆  How important are my kinks?

◆  Where do they fit into my identity as a human being?

◆  How might my life or happiness be affected (or not affected) if I weren't able to explore my kinks?

Understanding this can help you formulate a blueprint for how you want to incorporate kink into your life.

"For some people, kink is part of their sexuality. For others, it's just something they take part in," Rea Pearson, a sex-positive BACP-accredited counselor and relationship therapist, specializing in working with gender, sexuality, and relationship diversities, told me in an interview.

If your kinks are an essential component of your happiness and fulfillment, this isn't anything to be ashamed of. It's entirely valid. It's just a matter of figuring out a way to incorporate them into your sex life in a way that works for you—and possibly a current or future partner.

Feel free to save this bigger existential question on the importance of kink until later down the road. You don't need to have the answers yet. I only wanted to introduce it here so you could start to think about it as we unpack your desires.

## UNDERSTANDING THE EROTIC MIND

The first thing we have to do is understand exactly how the erotic mind *works* to fully explore it.

When I say, "exploring the erotic mind," I'm referring to the thoughts, memories, fantasies, activities, and so forth that turn you on. Understanding these elements is a big component of living your most authentic sexual life—and kinkiest life, too! Knowing what turns you on gives you "a map of your unique erotic landscape and, therefore, helps you choose the right sexual/romantic partner(s) for yourself, and be more likely to have great pleasurable experiences," Silva Neves, an accredited psychosexual and relationship psychotherapist (and creator of the highly popular "erotic mind" course at Beducated.com) told me in an interview.

### The first thing to unpack: How our sexual interests develop in the first place

We've gone pretty in-depth in previous chapters about how kinks and fetishes develop, but let's take a moment to break down the nuts and bolts of how all sexual interests develop for us wee humans. As we know, we're creative AF and our capacity for fantasy is wildly complex and expansive.

I've pointed to childhood as one possible origin for desires, but this is a bit reductive. "Our erotic mind is just as diverse as nature is," Neves explains. "The problem is that if sexual interests are part of the 'norm,' nobody questions them, but if they are unusual, people tend to think that it is because something went wrong in childhood." And that's just not the case. Fantasy and sexual interest can certainly develop out of childhood, but they also develop out of many other avenues and at different times in our lives. We have to think bigger, people!

"We like what we like," Cyndi Darnell, sex therapist and author of *Sex, When You Don't Feel Like It: The Truth About Mismatched Libido & Rediscovering Desire*, tells me. "No need for further analysis."

### The four cornerstones of the erotic mind*

Neves identifies four cornerstones of the erotic mind that are worth considering:

1. searching for power

2. overcoming ambivalence

3. longing and anticipation

4. violating prohibitions.

These are some of the root motivations behind why something

---

\*    The concept of the erotic mind was originally created by Jack Morin in his 1995 book, *The Erotic Mind*.

(real or fantasy) may take on sexual meaning. "Some people may find only one of those cornerstones of eroticism very erotically potent, while others might have two or three they find very arousing," he tells us. "Some may have none. But generally speaking, people will find some of their turn-on[s] enhanced when they come across one of [these] cornerstones." Exploring these cornerstones and considering how they may play into your fantasies can help you better understand yourself as a sexual being.

Are sexual desires and fantasies ever a cause for concern? The short answer: not really.

Some folx may think that their fantasies and/or sexual desires are problematic, but this isn't the case, generally speaking. "There is nothing 'wrong' [with] having fantasies, even if the fantasies are about things that are illegal," Neves says.

As triggering as this may be, there is a massive difference between *thinking* about something illegal and *acting* on something illegal. Fantasies are the wild, weird, often freaky AF creations of our incredibly rich imaginations. This content should be explored for better self-understanding, not shrouded in fear and shame. And this is especially true when we're talking about kink. Oftentimes, we self-censor because we believe our kinks are trauma-filled nightmares that make us bad people—but this just isn't the case. I promise you, you're completely normal and OK for having taboo sexual interests.

## UNDERSTANDING YOUR EROTIC MIND IS KEY TO REDUCING SHAME

Exploring your erotic mind can be a powerful tool for reducing shame. Why? Well, because we live in a sex-negative hellscape that doesn't encourage sexual exploration. It's radical and self-actualizing to subvert this narrative through the navigation of your sexual template.

What if you could reframe exploring your erotic mind as a way to get to know the real you, even with all the shadows and darker stuff? "Your erotic mind can be a place that illuminates more of who you are, especially the parts that you try to hide and don't like to admit are there," sexologist Lucy Rowett explains. "The human sexual subconscious is a very transgressive place, it's where we explore the taboo and what cannot be said, so embrace it." When we embrace our sexual selves, we embrace what it means to be a free human being.

OK! With all this juicy information locked and loaded, let's go even deeper and explore what you're into using the erotic mind as our jumping-off point. You'll also find an exercise at the end of the chapter that invites you to make a map of your erotic mind using peak sexual experiences. Here are three simple steps to unravel what you might be into.

## STEP 1: YES, NO, MAYBE LIST

You don't know what you don't know if you don't know it—you know? You might be kinky AF and still haven't fully explored the amazing, deliciously expansive kinks that are out there waiting for you. There are *so* many kinks and fetishes. The exact number would likely be impossible to fully quantify because the human mind is so endlessly creative and horny. But we shall try.

A great place to get started with discovering your kinks is by going through a list of possible options and thinking: "Is this something I'm into? Could I possibly be into this? Or is it a hell no?" Enter the Yes, No, Maybe list.

This is a list of the kinks and fetishes available for exploration—or at least, most of them. To use it, you go through the list systematically and for each option ask yourself: "Is this a Yes, a No, or a Maybe?" A maybe indicates that you aren't entirely sure if you're into it, but you might be willing to try it, or at least explore the possibility further.

Now, there are so many amazing Yes, No, Maybe lists out there, so if this book's list isn't doing it for you, you can always Google "Kinky Yes, No, Maybe list" and you're likely to find one that will do the job. I've personally read and recommended dozens of lists based on each client's needs in my clinical work, so this book's Yes, No, Maybe list is inspired by outside sources. For another fabulous kink option, I suggest Love N' Kink podcast's extensive list and educator Sunny Megatron's list. You can also check out more general non-kink lists from Scarleteen and Sex with Emily.

The Yes, No, Maybe list is meant to be used as a jumping-off point—as a way to get your creative juices flowing—hence why I'm calling it "Step 1." Whether you're 100 percent set on your kinks or have no idea what you want, this list can be helpful. It's all about learning more about yourself.

At this point in the book, you've already reviewed consent safety checklists and sexual health safety checklists, so you should feel pretty solid about these foundations—they are essential to practicing kink safely. We're now ready to build upon these first solid layers by introducing actual kink play scenarios and acts within this safe context.

To get cracking, pop down to the end of this chapter where I've provided a worksheet to fill out. There are additional prompts to help you suss out your limits within each kink. For example, is there a body part you do not want to be touched? Or perhaps there is a word or phrase you do not want a partner to use? Adding these in and writing them down can help make kink more accessible because you can learn to engage with it in a way that feels safe for you.

I've indicated "giving" and "receiving" as another means of whittling down what you want from each kink. For example, if you put "yes" next to bondage, would you like to be tied up or to do the tying? If the answer is both, feel free to circle both giving and receiving. Considering this is a good way to start to unpick how you picture your role within this kink dynamic, which can, in turn, help you start to flesh out what the scene might ideally look like for you.

We'll come back to the Yes, No, Maybe list in Chapter 14, where we bring your partner into the fun.

## STEP 2: USING EROTIC CONTENT FOR INSPIRATION

Using porn and other erotic content is such an amazing way to start exploring different kinds of kink play and figuring out what gets you going. Since you've dutifully filled out your Yes, No, Maybe list, you now have some concepts, roles, and types of play you might want to explore in the fantasy realm.

It's important that when we're choosing erotic content, you're looking for content that isn't, well, shit. Mainstream porn (think free tube sites) is a form of highly stylized entertainment that is geared toward cis-het men. There are all kinds of questionable practices going on behind the scenes as well as in them. If you've ever watched a mainstream gang bang scene, you'll probably know what I'm talking about. There is a lens placed on men dominating women, punish-f*cking them, with questionable consent (if consent is present at all).

Which is why we want to be sure that what we're consuming is ethical. Now, you might be thinking: "There's an ethical way for me to watch a woman be turned into a human chandelier in a rope harness and be anally penetrated that is considered above board?" Yes, this is correct!

With the rise of ethically made porn, stricter standards (standardized, fair pay for actors, STI testing, collaborations over scripts and scenes that take the actors' boundaries into account, and so forth, just more human respect) are (slowly) being implemented in smaller indie studios. And this is super important for everyone involved—from the viewer, to the crew, to the actors.

Why is this important for you? Because you want to be sure that the kink content you're consuming is high quality, with everyone enjoying themselves and practicing safely. Porn is not education—so don't take it as a substitute for workshops, classes, or reading this book (hi!). This is meant to serve as inspiration.

OK, where do I find good ethically made material?

## 1. CrashPad Series

"CrashPad Series is a queer, non-binary, and female-focused studio with authentic, playful, genuine connections and sexual expression with a diverse array of body types, presentations, identities, and expressions," sex educator Lorrae Bradbury told me in an interview. "They cast real-world couples having the sex they truly enjoy at their comfort level, complete with safer sex, communication, aftercare, and the genuine laughter and silliness that can often be part of sex."

## 2. Royal Fetish Films

King and Jet Setting Jasmine run Royal Fetish Films and are setting a high industry standard in ethical porn. Their content is inclusive, beautifully made, and incredibly kinky.

## 3. Bellesa

Bellesa is free-to consume, curated porn. It's porn for women and femmes, made by women and femmes. There is something for everyone, and kink certainly abounds.

## 4. Cheex

"Cheex includes carefully curated erotic films from independent artists and production companies, plus erotic audio stories and educational resources with articles and interviews around sexual wellness and pleasure," Bradbury says.

## 5. SPIT

According to Bradbury, "SPIT incorporates photos, audio erotica, and videos from naked storytime to partnered play, highlighting diverse sexual expression that takes you on an authentic journey through desire and exploration."

## 6. Erika Lust

Erika Lust is one of the top producers of ethical porn in the biz. If you're looking for movie-quality smut, this is the place.

### 7. Dipsea

Dipsea is an audioerotica app that can be a fabulous option for anyone who doesn't enjoy visual representations of sex. It has countless steamy stories.

### 8. Afterglow

Brand-new on the scene is Afterglow, the newest star on the ethical porn horizon. They have amazing options for everyone and anyone.

You can also subscribe to OnlyFans creators that you particularly like. This is a great way to support your local sex workers—and find content that you want to see!

## STEP 3: USING JOURNALING

Thus far, I've put some journal prompts at the end of each chapter, but I've brought them into the fold for Chapter 9 because journaling is such a fantastic tool for figuring out what it is you're into. You've done the Yes, No, Maybe list, and you've explored some erotic content, so hopefully the creative juices are flowing.

### Time to reflect

1. Consider the four cornerstones of the erotic mind we discussed earlier. Try asking yourself these questions: What is my first sexual memory? What fantasies do I have? What is my favorite sexual act? Reflect on this.

2. Consider your Yes, No, Maybe list and reflect on the following: Did anything on the list surprise you? Scare you? Repulse you? Turn you on? Where do you think these feelings come from?

Do any memories or experiences come to mind? Think about any strong emotional or physical reactions you experienced and reflect on them below.

3. Consider your exploration into erotic content and reflect on the following: Did you find anything you enjoyed? If yes, reflect on why you enjoyed this content. Think about what it was about the content that was so enticing. Was it the acts themselves? The power dynamics? The tools used? Was it the words the actors were using? Who did you relate to in the scene? Did you discover anything about yourself and your interests?

**AGONY AUNT QUESTION AND ANSWER:**
**I want to sub. Is that weird?**

Q *Dear Auntie Gigi,*

*A bit of background on me: I'm a dominant person in real life. I'm a cis straight man who has a high-powered career and a lot of responsibilities. I really enjoy this aspect of my life, though it can be overwhelming. Here is the thing: I think I want to be a submissive in the bedroom. I think I also want to wear costumes, but maybe not. I have no idea if this is normal or if a partner would even be OK with this. Every woman I've been with has been quite submissive and expects me to take charge in the bedroom. I'm able to comply and I do enjoy it, but I just have a real feeling that I want something different. Am I a superfreak for maybe wanting to be submissive? How do I figure out if this is something I actually want?*

*Unsure sub*

A Dear Unsure sub,

Believe it or not, this possible desire to take on a more submissive role in the bedroom is entirely natural. While people who want to sub have all kinds of backgrounds and levels of power in their daily lives, the desire to take on a different role from the one you're used to in your everyday life makes a lot of sense.

Let's think about this for a second. You're someone who has a ton of responsibilities and pressures to cope with. While it's great that you find joy in your life, this amount of stress can certainly take its toll both mentally and physically. It's just a lot of shit to deal with. As a submissive in the bedroom, you would get the opportunity to relinquish control to someone else. You wouldn't have to worry about anything at all—you'd simply trust in your Dom to handle everything. It would be an escape from the pressures of your life in a safe and contained way. When we break it down like this, doesn't it sound appealing? It's a way to take a break without any risk of it impacting your real life.

So, are you a superfreak? Not at all. You're perfectly normal for wanting this. Kink offers us an opportunity to explore power dynamics to obtain an experience we desire. Wanting to be submissive, regardless of your gender or life circumstances, is normal.

Since you're unsure if this is something you want, I'd encourage you to start exploring erotic content that aligns with these desires. Reflect on how it makes you feel. I also always recommend journaling, as it gives us a chance to get our thoughts down on paper and see things more clearly. Sometimes we want things to happen in real life, and other times we want things to remain in our fantasies. Understanding where you fall on this spectrum is important because it will give you information about how you want this to fit into your life.

As for costumes, consider what kinds of costumes you'd want to try. You can even purchase a couple online and try them on in private. Remember to be gentle with yourself. Instead of judging your interests and wallowing in shame, look at them with empathy and curiosity. There is absolutely nothing wrong with wanting to dress up as a sissy maid in one of those classic black and white sexy dresses, for example. Society likes to demonize straight men for wanting anything that falls outside of the binary of what we socially consider "masculine." This is harmful. There is nothing wrong with wanting to explore things on the gender spectrum during kink play. I assure you, there is nothing wrong with you. Human beings are creative in the best way possible. It's fantastic that you have such an expansive imagination.

Explore your desires before bringing them to a partner. You want to be sure you're feeling secure in what you want before you invite someone else in.

I hope this helps.

Auntie Gigi XOXO

# EXERCISES

## EXERCISE 1: Mapping the erotic mind

(Adapted from Jack Morin's work in his book *The Erotic Mind*, 1995)

You're going to have to bring out the drawing skills now because we are about to make a map! If drawing and pictures are not your thing—due to neurodivergence or just generally not enjoying it—feel free to list things in any format that works for you.

**Step 1:** Take time to scan and consider your sexual history—this can be both in fantasy and reality. Choose a peak sexual experience. This is one where you felt really connected, really turned on, or fulfilled. A peak sexual experience is one that you truly, truly enjoyed (even if you're afraid to admit it). Put this memory in the center of your map and circle it.

**Step 2:** Draw a circle around the center circle. In this circle, start writing down what led you to this sexual experience. Recall the surrounding details. What were you wearing? Who were you with? What environment were you in? Do you recall smells, sounds, or other sensory experiences?

**Step 3:** Draw another circle around the map so far—you should have a circle, within a circle, within a circle now. In this area, write down details of the experience itself. What happened? What details stand out to you? What acts were involved? What did your partner do or say (if a partner was present)? Do you recall smells, sounds, or other sensory experiences?

**Step 4:** Draw a final circle around the outside of the circles you have. Start writing down all the qualities of this memory that you want to experience more of. What stands out to you? Try to get as specific as possible.

**Step 5:** Below your map, reflect on the positive qualities that you pulled out. Why are they enticing? What makes them so appealing? Why do you want to experience more of them? What do you think this tells you about yourself and your desires?

Hold on to this map for future use, and feel free to go back to this exercise anytime you want to understand a sexual memory (and why you loved it) more closely. Repeat as desired.

## EXERCISE 2: Yes, No, Maybe list

**Step 1:** Circle the answer that feels most right for you.

**Step 2:** If you're unsure what a certain item or act on the list is, refer to the glossary. And if it isn't there, just Google [insert item/act] kink definition.

**Dominance**

Yes No Maybe Giving Receiving

**Submission**

Yes No Maybe Giving Receiving

**Sadism**

Yes No Maybe Giving Receiving

**Masochism**

Yes No Maybe Giving Receiving

**Voyeurism**

Yes No Maybe Giving Receiving

**Exhibitionism**

Yes No Maybe Giving Receiving

**Anal play** (rimming)

Yes No Maybe Giving Receiving

**Anal play** (prostate play)

Yes No Maybe Giving Receiving

**Anal play** (using butt plugs)

Yes No Maybe Giving Receiving

**Anal play** (anal penetration, including with a dildo)

Yes No Maybe Giving Receiving

**Age play**

Yes No Maybe Giving Receiving

**Bondage** (using rope)

Yes No Maybe Giving Receiving

**Bondage** (using handcuffs, velcro restraints, etc.)
Yes No Maybe Giving Receiving

**Cock torture**
Yes No Maybe Giving Receiving

**Clit and vulva torture**
Yes No Maybe Giving Receiving

**Using cages**
Yes No Maybe Giving Receiving

**Ball gag** (or other form of gag)
Yes No Maybe Giving Receiving

**Orgasm control play**
Yes No Maybe Giving Receiving

**Forced orgasms**
Yes No Maybe Giving Receiving

**Edging**
Yes No Maybe Giving Receiving

**Orgasm denial**
Yes No Maybe Giving Receiving

**Permission to orgasm**
Yes No Maybe Giving Receiving

**Pegging**
Yes No Maybe Giving Receiving

**Masturbation using sex toys**
Yes No Maybe Giving Receiving

**Mutual masturbation**
Yes No Maybe Giving Receiving

**Masturbating your partner**
Yes No Maybe Giving Receiving

**Nipple clamps**
Yes No Maybe Giving Receiving

**Clitoral clamp**
Yes No Maybe Giving Receiving

**Chastity belt**
Yes No Maybe Giving Receiving

**Forced abstinence**
Yes No Maybe Giving Receiving

**Tickling**
Yes No Maybe Giving Receiving

**Spanking** (using a bare hand)
Yes No Maybe Giving Receiving

**Spanking** (using a paddle, flogger, or other implements)
Yes No Maybe Giving Receiving

**Spanking** (using household items like a wooden spoon or spatula)
Yes No Maybe Giving Receiving

**Strap-on play**

Yes  No  Maybe  Giving  Receiving

**Impact play** (using floggers, crops, and other implements)

Yes  No  Maybe  Giving  Receiving

**Impact play** (slapping or hitting with hands)

Yes  No  Maybe  Giving  Receiving

**Rule following**

Yes  No  Maybe  Giving  Receiving

**Setting rules**

Yes  No  Maybe  Giving  Receiving

**Punishments** (such as sitting in a chair, having privileges removed, being caged, or name-calling)

Yes  No  Maybe  Giving  Receiving

**Boot licking**

Yes  No  Maybe  Giving  Receiving

**Slapping**

Yes  No  Maybe  Giving  Receiving

**Nipple torture**

Yes  No  Maybe  Giving  Receiving

**Hair pulling**

Yes  No  Maybe  Giving  Receiving

**Wax play**

Yes  No  Maybe  Giving  Receiving

**Wartenberg Wheel** (wheel with spikes)

Yes  No  Maybe  Giving  Receiving

**Vibrators during play**

Yes  No  Maybe  Giving  Receiving

**Dildos during play**

Yes  No  Maybe  Giving  Receiving

**DD/lg play**

Yes  No  Maybe  Giving  Receiving

**Cock rings**

Yes  No  Maybe  Giving  Receiving

**Oral sex**

Yes  No  Maybe  Giving  Receiving

**Handjob/fingering**

Yes  No  Maybe  Giving  Receiving

**Sex in public**

Yes  No  Maybe  Giving  Receiving

**Threesome**

Yes  No  Maybe  Giving  Receiving

**Temperature play**

Yes  No  Maybe  Giving  Receiving

**Gang bangs**

Yes  No  Maybe  Giving  Receiving

**Group sex**

Yes  No  Maybe  Giving  Receiving

**Cuckold play**

Yes  No  Maybe  Giving  Receiving

**Sexting**

Yes  No  Maybe  Giving  Receiving

**Sensory play**

Yes  No  Maybe  Giving  Receiving

**Phone sex**

Yes  No  Maybe  Giving  Receiving

**Pain play**

Yes  No  Maybe  Giving  Receiving

**Video sex**

Yes  No  Maybe  Giving  Receiving

**Massage**

Yes  No  Maybe  Giving  Receiving

**Biting**

Yes  No  Maybe  Giving  Receiving

**Licking**

Yes  No  Maybe  Giving  Receiving

**Sensory deprivation**

Yes  No  Maybe  Giving  Receiving

**Collar**

Yes  No  Maybe  Giving  Receiving

**Cuffs**

Yes  No  Maybe  Giving  Receiving

**Latex clothing**

Yes  No  Maybe  Giving  Receiving

**Sex swing**

Yes  No  Maybe  Giving  Receiving

**Sex wedge**

Yes  No  Maybe  Giving  Receiving

**Breath play**

Yes  No  Maybe  Giving  Receiving

**Knife play**

Yes  No  Maybe  Giving  Receiving

**Blood play**

Yes  No  Maybe  Giving  Receiving

**Golden shower**

Yes  No  Maybe  Giving  Receiving

**Scat play**

Yes  No  Maybe  Giving  Receiving

**Pet play** (puppy play, kitty play, pony play, etc.)

Yes  No  Maybe  Giving  Receiving

**Praise kink**

Yes No Maybe Giving Receiving

**St. Andrew's cross**

Yes No Maybe Giving Receiving

**Spanking bench**

Yes No Maybe Giving Receiving

Short answer prompts:

♦   Sexual acts that are off-limits for me:

. . . . . . . . . . . . . . . . . . . . . . . . . . . . . . . . . . . . . . . . . . . . . . . .

. . . . . . . . . . . . . . . . . . . . . . . . . . . . . . . . . . . . . . . . . . . . . . . .

♦   Body parts that are off-limits for me:

. . . . . . . . . . . . . . . . . . . . . . . . . . . . . . . . . . . . . . . . . . . . . . . .

. . . . . . . . . . . . . . . . . . . . . . . . . . . . . . . . . . . . . . . . . . . . . . . .

♦   Body parts that are of particular interest to me:

. . . . . . . . . . . . . . . . . . . . . . . . . . . . . . . . . . . . . . . . . . . . . . . .

. . . . . . . . . . . . . . . . . . . . . . . . . . . . . . . . . . . . . . . . . . . . . . . .

♦   Words and phrases I do not want to use or hear from a partner:

. . . . . . . . . . . . . . . . . . . . . . . . . . . . . . . . . . . . . . . . . . . . . . . .

. . . . . . . . . . . . . . . . . . . . . . . . . . . . . . . . . . . . . . . . . . . . . . . .

♦   Words and phrases I do want to use or to hear from my partner:

. . . . . . . . . . . . . . . . . . . . . . . . . . . . . . . . . . . . . . . . . . . . . . . .

. . . . . . . . . . . . . . . . . . . . . . . . . . . . . . . . . . . . . . . . . . . . . . . .

◆   I need extra support or care around certain sexual or erotic acts,
    and those are:

    . . . . . . . . . . . . . . . . . . . . . . . . . . . . . . . . . . . . . . . . . . . . . . . . . .

    . . . . . . . . . . . . . . . . . . . . . . . . . . . . . . . . . . . . . . . . . . . . . . . . . .

## EXERCISE 3: Two grounding exercises for anxious folx

Going through your erotic mind can be a bit overwhelming. If you've
found this to be the case, try these two simple exercises to ground
yourself and feel more present. Always check in with your mental state
and be sure to take care of your well-being. Feel free to use this at
any time throughout the rest of the book.

### BOX BREATHING

You're going to breathe in a box formation. Take a deep breath in for
a count of four. Hold it for a count of four. Breath out for a count of
four. Repeat this three to five times until you feel calm. This exercise
is useful because it resets the nervous system and is quite easy to
remember in times of distress.

### THE FIVE SENSES TECHNIQUE

This exercise is incredibly popular in psychotherapy because it helps
bring us back into the moment when we're feeling heightened. It
breaks the stress cycle by forcing you to pay attention to your sur-
roundings. This is essential when you're anxious and lost in your head.

I've simplified the exercise to make it as straightforward as
possible. Wherever you are, stop, take a deep breath, and name
the following:

◆   three things you can see

- three things you can hear

- three things you can smell

- three things you can touch

- three things you can taste (*Note:* This one can be challenging, so if you can only name one or two, that's completely fine).

Here's an example of how to do this: I'm currently sitting at my writing desk on a warm spring day.

- Three things I can see: my hanging spider plant, a mug full of pens, and my black Moleskine notebook on my desk.

- Three things I can hear: the sound of traffic outside my open window, the sound of keys clicking as I type, and voices down on the street.

- Three things I can smell: my coffee, the vague scent of spring, and my skin cream as I bring my hand to my face.

- Three things I can touch: My phone sitting next to me, my coffee mug, and the edge of my desk.

- Three things I can taste: coffee, air as I suck in, and my electrolyte drink.

## Chapter 9 recap

In Chapter 9, we laid out a plan for figuring out what you're into, with some tangible ways to get there. We explored how the erotic mind works and how to explore it with a mapping exercise.

We then looked at three simple steps for starting to suss out what you desire:

- Yes, No, Maybe lists (with an accompanying exercise)
- erotic content
- journaling.

I provided an Agony Aunt letter to illustrate the advice and guidance I would give a real-life person who was interested in exploring their submissive desires, and how to decide how they'd want to incorporate them into their life.

Hopefully, you feel equipped to use the tools provided in this chapter to whittle down what it is you want out of kink and how you might like to explore.

# 10

## DOM? SUB? TOP? BOTTOM? SWITCH? HOW TO EMBRACE YOUR AUTHENTIC KINK IDENTITY

**What you'll find in this chapter:**

➜ The spectrum of kink identities and how to find where you fall.

➜ How to be a good Dom.

➜ How to be a good sub.

➜ What about switches?

➜ Agony Aunt questions and answers.

➜ Exercises.

## THE DOM TO SUB SPECTRUM

**C** **ontrary to what you might believe,** Dom and sub roles aren't black and white. Instead of thinking of Dominance and submission as definitive labels, we can think of them as falling on a spectrum. On one side is a person who is 100 percent Dom through and through, and on the other is a person who is an all-out, balls-to-the-wall submissive. Most people will fall somewhere along the spectrum of full Dom and full sub. Considering it in this way can help you start to pick and choose the qualities that work for you and your identity around being Dom, sub, or switch.

Yes, it isn't super clear-cut, and I'm sorry it can't be easier, but such is life.

Within this spectrum are a whole host of different kinds of Doms, subs, and switches. We've looked at quite a few throughout the book so far.

| Sub | Switch | Dom |
|---|---|---|

Some common Dom archetypes:

- Mommy/Daddy/Caretaker
- Goddess/God
- Master/Mistress
- Pet owner.

Some common sub archetypes:

- slave
- pet
- brat
- baby/little girl/little boy.

Categories can be helpful when you're wading into the unknown waters of kink play for the first time, but as sex educator and spicy content creator Alice Lovegood wrote in a blog post on finding your kink persona, how your kink identity manifests is entirely subjective. There are broad categories, but every Dom, sub, and switch will show up differently:

> These "labels" can be helpful in creating an identity, or learning about someone, as well as connecting with others that feel similarly, but the way one person Dominates, and how another brats or submits, and the ways they exchange power, reward, punish and more, are all individual to that unique dynamic and should be discussed and decided as such. This is simply a learning tool and not a copy–paste application.

On the spectrum of Dom to sub, there are also those fun topsy-turvy labels of Top and bottom. Yes, pun intended. You might, for example, identify as a Service Top—someone who provides pleasure, stimulation, etc., based on the sub's needs and desires. A Service Top acts in service of the sub, rather than from a place of dominance. Within this identity, you may or may not also call yourself a Dom. It truly is a choose-your-own-adventure. You might also remember the example of Shibari. Rope Tops may be doing the "doing," but they don't always see their role as being dominant.

The long and short of it is you can be a Dom, sub, or switch in any way you want to be. It's about figuring out what works for you. As Lovegood told me in an interview:

> People can get into a mindset of taking kink and BDSM very seriously and have this fear of getting things wrong but sex, kink

and BDSM should be treated like an adult playground. It's an opportunity to play, explore, and have fun.

You may very well try one role and think, "Nope. This is not for me, mate!" and that is perfectly OK. It's through the lens of curiosity that we get to discover who we want to be in kink.

Lovegood shared this truly delightful metaphor:

> We would never find our favorite meal if we didn't try different dishes; kinks are like the ingredients. You know you hate Marmite and you know you're not going to like a dish with a Marmite base, but if you like chicken and spicy flavors then the chicken fajita dish might be worth a go; maybe it will become a new favorite staple, or maybe an unexpected flavor will leave a sour taste in your mouth; maybe you can take that one ingredient out and adapt the dish to your tastes—you won't know until you try.

## HOW TO BE A GOOD DOM

Being a good Dom starts with asking yourself the fundamental question: *Why is being a Dom appealing to me?* "Being a good Dominant is a mix of natural inclination, self-awareness, and ongoing growth," says Nia Jane, a psychosexual therapist specializing in kink. Throughout this book, you've done a lot of journaling around your desires and fantasies. So, for the baby Doms, what is it about Domming that you find so interesting? The power it offers? Being a leader? Taking someone on a physical and emotional journey? Sadism? Control? There are no wrong answers because it's really about figuring out what you want at your core.

A good Dom has "typically already done a good bit of introspection—enough to know what they're into, and have a solid understanding of power dynamics and why it all appeals," Nia Jane says. We have to understand the "why" before we can get into the "how."

Being a good Dom has much less to do with brandishing a whip with reckless abandon and more to do with fully immersing yourself in a character. It's possible to have a Dom/sub scene without any gear at all, as long as both parties are fully committed to the dynamic. Authenticity is the name of the game. I think knowing this helps us understand that kink truly is for anyone and everyone. It isn't about having a personalized dungeon with a bespoke spanking bench and a St. Andrew's cross—it's about investing in your character and embracing the Dom within.

And remember: You're allowed to flirt with the idea of being a Dom and try it out, even if you're not entirely sure if this is right for you. Give it a go and see how you feel about it. Check in with yourself and your partner to assess how you're getting on with this role. Being a good Dom is a lot about confidence, but that confidence doesn't just materialize out of nowhere. It has to be cultivated—and that takes patience and practice!

## The top five qualities that make a good Dom

### Learning your skills

"If I were to identify one trait that showed a good Dom from a bad Dom, it would be a Dom that takes responsibility to educate themselves, learn and develop," Lovegood tells me. And this also includes continuous learning. Like any skill, becoming a good Dom takes time and effort. It requires practice, which is ongoing and never-ending (in the best possible way).

Skills for Doms:

- understanding sexual health and safety

- developing skills based on the activities you're engaging in (e.g., learning how to use a flogger, understanding "no go" zones of the body, learning to tie ropes)

- building a collection of gear (e.g., having your own ropes/floggers/crops/collars)

- having safety gear on hand (e.g., shears for cutting rope, first-aid kit, ice packs)

- understanding safe words and boundaries.

### Boundary setting

As a Dominant, your job is to make sure that the sub's boundaries are respected. Reed Amber, an OnlyFans creator, kink enthusiast, and co-host of the Come Curious podcast, told me that a Dom not only needs to be able to hold the boundaries of their submissive, but needs to be crystal f-ing clear about their own boundaries. Just because you're the Dom, doesn't mean you have to do something you don't want to do just because your submissive partner is frothing-at-the-mouth horny for it. Sit down and have a conversation about boundaries—and make a commitment to adhere to them.

Here is where the "enthusiastic maybe" comes into play: You might not know exactly if something is your cup of tea, but you're willing to give it a go. Be open about your "maybes" and discuss action plans if things don't go as intended.

For instance, perhaps you haven't spanked someone before, but you think you might be into it. Discuss with the sub where and how they would like to be spanked. Is it with hands, a flogger, a crop? Do they enjoy spanking on their bum, thighs, or both? Have a safe word in place (which can be used by both of you), should you decide you're not a fan after all.

## Attunement

A key ingredient in effective Domming is a little thing called empathy. You have to be able to stay in emotional contact with the sub to accurately read the erotic situation. "They need an ability to read someone's body language, and they need to leave their ego at the door; they cannot allow themselves to get charged up and act irresponsibly," Lovegood says. "It takes a lot of control to Dom well and with care, and above all the sub needs to trust and feel safe with you."

## Creating a clear aesthetic

While not every Dom needs to take their Dom character to the point of dressing up, setting up a dungeon space, and becoming a different person, it can be a great way to get into your role. Reed Amber says that being a good Dom is about embodying the Dom you want to be. You have to step into the character.

> You want to create this air of power and approachability. With that power is knowing yourself and being careful and looking good, kind of exuding a character or a persona that you want to be when you are being Dom. That could literally be a dominant suit or it could be leather, or it could be a Dom that revolves around the idea of cults and religion. But having that sort of clear view of how you want to look—especially because clothing has such a huge part to play in getting into character and getting into the scene.

### Clear and ongoing communication

If you want to Dom, you have to learn how to effectively communicate. This means being able to speak up when something doesn't feel right, adhering to safe words and boundaries, and regularly checking in with your sub to ensure everyone is feeling safe and secure. Lovegood says that you don't have to break character to communicate effectively as a Dom. Learning to communicate while staying in your Dom energy is a learned skill that can be developed over time. Here are some spicy examples, courtesy of Lovegood, on how you might go about this.

- "Sub, tell me where we are in intensity. I shouldn't have to ask you."

- "Shall we find a five intensity level? I want to see what your pretty ass can take so I can take you to the edge."

- "Show me how you want to be touched. Yes, there's a good girl."

- "Use your words, beg me."

## WHY EVERY GOOD DOM SHOULD TRY SUBBING...OR SHOULD THEY?

You can't really escape the "how to be a good Dom" conversation without addressing the notion that every good Dom needs to try subbing if they truly want to be a good Dom. This is a rather spicy take within the kink community.

Do you need to try subbing to be an effective Dom? The answer: maybe and maybe not.

Trying a sub role is a great way to learn what the sub is

experiencing, which can help you craft your skills. You're going to have a broader understanding of punishments, spankings, and submission if you have been a submissive.

Because being a good Dom requires a massive amount of attunement and empathy, the question becomes: How can you be attuned to a sub if you don't know what they're going through? Most of the kink enthusiasts I chatted to while researching this book told me they wouldn't consider subbing for someone who hadn't tried subbing themselves. And you know what? That's fair. We all get to decide what and who we are and are not willing to engage with. I'd suggest always asking a Dom (or sub) if they've tried the other role and how those experiences were for them. Reed Amber says that sub experience is a must for her, and if a Dom hasn't been a sub, it's a red flag. "For me, it creates massive warning bells that they are maybe not actually comfortable being vulnerable because being submissive is an extremely vulnerable space." As a Dom, you should be willing to put yourself in that place, too. "The person that you're playing with should be a part of that learning process. Even if it's not something that sexually turns you on. It still is an important part of understanding how you make a submissive feel."

However, Nia Jane says we can't be out here painting with broad strokes and making big claims. Yes, trying out subbing can be super helpful—and perhaps quite humbling (in a good way, hopefully)—but this is just not going to work for everyone. If you really, truly do not want to sub, it probably won't be the most cash-money experience for you. "Pushing someone into a role they're really not comfortable with just for the sake of understanding the 'other side'? Not ideal," she says. "A strong D-type is just likely to find the whole experience frustrating and forced, which doesn't benefit anyone. And if the idea is that the submissive-leaning partner then takes the Dominant role, well, they're probably going to feel equally uncomfortable with that."

If you're super down to clown in Dom Town, but the idea of subbing repulses you, it's important to ask yourself: Why? Why am I so averse to this? Because getting into the weeds of that distaste can also serve as an eye-opening experience that can highlight certain biases. For example, if you're a cis-man who only wants to Dom, is it because you see subbing as a feminine or less-than role? Or perhaps your ego is threatened? These questions are not about passing judgment but rather are tools to help us understand ourselves better.

What it comes down to is this: Most subs won't want to play with a Dom who has never tried subbing. Does this mean you have to try subbing? No. You don't have to do anything you don't want to do. But keep in mind that this might impact who you get to play with—personal agency, and all that.

**AGONY AUNT QUESTION AND ANSWER: My partner wants me to Dom them. Now what?**

Q *Dear Auntie Gigi,*

*My partner (F32) and I (M38) have been together for nearly seven years. We've had a great sex life for most of our relationship, other than a brief period after our son was born three years ago. We've never really done anything "kinky" before. It's not something I've thought a lot about. We have a good sexual connection, and I thought we were on the same page. We have good, normal sex, and we both experience a lot of pleasure.*

*I always make sure she's satisfied. But here's the issue: My partner has recently come to me and said she's always wanted to try kink. She really wants me to Dom her and to start bringing this stuff into our regular sex life. I do think I'm open to the idea of giving this a try, although I'm pretty worried I'll be terrible at it. I've never done anything like this before. So, where do we begin? Is this even a realistic proposition if I'm nearly 40 and have never even so much as spanked a girlfriend before?*

*Anxious Wannabe Dom*

A Dear Anxious Wannabe Dom,

First, congratulations on this new and exciting journey! An openness and willingness to explore are the true key ingredients that make a journey into kink possible. So, you're almost 40 and are afraid kink might be off the table. Where on earth did you get this message? You're never too old to try kink. It doesn't matter if you're 19, 25, or 85—you can give kink a go. Yes, you're going to be a beginner, and your skills will take time to develop, but that does not in any way mean you are excluded from the kink club.

OK, now that we have this self-inflicted ageism out of the way, let's talk about getting started on your journey into embracing your identity as a Dom.

First, it's important to get clear on how *you* feel about this, rather than how you want to feel about it, because it's something your partner wants to do. It's great that you're open to giving being a Dom a try, but finding out if this role is authentic for you will help both of you have better experiences. Kink is so much better when both people are actually enjoying themselves, rather than half-heartedly engaging because they want to please their partner. With that being said, you may not *love* Domming, but discover you're happy to do it if your partner likes it. As long as both of you are comfortable with this dynamic, you can make it work.

So, is this appealing to you? What about it might be intriguing? What kind of Dom do you see yourself being? Start building your own fantasies around this. Read some erotic kink stories, watch some kink-positive porn (I have some great recommendations in Chapter 9), and journal.

Next, have an open and honest conversation with your partner. What is she envisioning for this Dom experience? What kinds of fantasies does she have? This can be a great opportunity to start getting the lusty fires burning, as well as a chance to collaborate on the scene. Remember, just because this is your partner's idea does not mean you have to do everything she wants. It should be a scene where both of your desires and fantasies can be explored in a way that feels safe and fun for both of you. Talk about your fantasies, get some inspiration, and enjoy yourselves. Sometimes all it takes is inspiration from someone, whether it be from yourself or the porn you're watching, to unlock someone's inner Dominant. Don't forget that these conversations need to be done with empathy and curiosity, rather than judgment. Turning toward your partner with openness can make all the difference.

I'd recommend either starting without complex gear or utilizing some homemade toys to begin. For instance, if you're exploring bondage, use a T-shirt or scarf as restraints. This way, you have a chance to practice without all the pressure of investing in expensive equipment.

Learn your stuff together—take a kink workshop, watch some YouTube tutorials, or read a book written by a qualified kink practitioner. Resources are only a Google away. You want to get clear on how to do certain acts safely before trying them. I have a few of my favorites at the end of the book in the "resources" section, too.

Take things really, really slowly. I mean, seriously. This might all be very exciting, but you don't know what you're doing yet, so give yourself grace. You may not know how you feel about this type of play once you take it from inside your head out into real life. You can start with simple acts of dominance like pinning your partner's wrists above their head during sex. As you feel more comfortable, you'll feel more at ease with pushing the boundaries.

Always remember to check in and see how both you and your partner are feeling before, during, and after sex.

Remember that sex and kink should be fun. We don't need to take ourselves so entirely seriously all the time, you know? This is an adventure that the two of you are embarking on together. Go slowly, take your time, let the awkwardness happen if it happens. We're all just trying our best.

XOXO Auntie Gigi

## HOW TO BE A GOOD SUB

If you want to be a sub, the first question to ask yourself is: *Why do I want to be a sub? What is it about being a sub that feels enticing to me?* Nia Jane says that Dom and sub are two sides of the same kinky coin—and so many of the same rules of effective Domming apply to effective subbing, though often inversely. "Submission is a gift that comes with a beautiful vulnerability, so it's important to think about what you need from a Dom to feel safe and secure," she says. "Consider your emotional needs, potential triggers, and how you'll navigate those tricky spots. Recognize your strengths and also the areas where you might need to do some work."

It's really all about trial and error in different kinds of play to discover what you are and are not into. And for that to work, trust is essential. This doesn't mean your partner needs to be a master Dominant before you can try submission; it just means you have to already have a foundation of trust to play safely. "Remember, sub does not = doormat! No one has the right to demand anything from you until you've agreed to it. Keep an eye out for red flags and keep your safety at the forefront always," Nia Jane adds.

## WHAT DOES BEING A SUB LOOK LIKE TO YOU?

Nia Jane says that while you don't have to fit into a limiting box, "it helps to figure out what styles of submission you vibe with—whether it's bratty, slave, little etc., whether you like things high or low protocol, and any other aspects that are really important to you." High protocol refers to more structured scenes and dynamics, whereas low protocol is more built around the Dom/sub dynamic, rather than the scene itself.

Some common sub archetypes:

◆ brat

◆ slave

◆ little girl/little boy/little/baby

◆ pet.

For Nia Jane, submission is all about working with her personality traits and desire for protocol:

> For me personally, my submissiveness is deeply intertwined with my service-oriented nature and a preference for high protocol dynamics. I thrive in a lifestyle-oriented, "24/7" dynamic where my submission extends beyond the bedroom and gets integrated into all the little aspects of daily life. I also have a very playful and bratty side, which adds an element of spontaneity and fun to the dynamic!

There is no one-size-fits-all (just like with Dominance!). Every single submissive is going to step into their submission differently. In a way, this subjective interpretation of the different D/s roles is incredibly liberating. You can explore power dynamics, scenes, and different forms of play in ways that feel completely authentic to you. You're not some cookie-cutter sub—you're a unique sub with your own playbook. While this might sound a bit intimidating, I would suggest reframing it as thinking: *There is no wrong way to do it*. You're only subbing wrong if you're being unsafe with your play, aren't respecting boundaries, are doing things you don't want to be doing, or aren't communicating effectively. It may sound bizarre, but it really is that simple.

# THE TOP FIVE QUALITIES THAT MAKE A GOOD SUB

## Authenticity

We often think of being a sub as being a character, and while this idea does have merit, it doesn't paint the whole picture. Yes, stepping into a role you've created is a big part of it, but it's really about the *authenticity* of that role. Being a truly amazing sub is being able to step into your sub self completely, shedding parts of your real-life self and bringing in parts of that self that align. Now, this does take time, confidence, and patience—but it's completely possible. The more you engage in scenes and kink play that feel right to you, the easier it becomes to melt into your sub character and embrace it fully. No one likes a half-hearted Dom, just as no one likes a lukewarm sub.

## Understanding your boundaries

Knowing your boundaries is essential when you're subbing because you're giving control to another person. Reed Amber says she won't even consider playing with a sub who says, "I don't have boundaries. Just do whatever you want to me." I completely agree with this. That sounds very much like a one-way ticket to getting deeply traumatized. Do not do this. You have to be able to effectively communicate what you do and don't want. Otherwise, Reed Amber says you're giving too much responsibility to a Dom, which can lead to things being pushed too far and making people feel unsafe or uncomfortable. Since you're new to subbing, you might not know your boundaries quite yet, which means you have to be ready to pull your safe word if something doesn't feel right for you. It's all about effective communication. Reed Amber adds that this may involve needing to break character in a scene.

## Clear and ongoing communication

Speaking of communication, having concise, clear, and ongoing communication is a must. This means being able to check in throughout a scene to let your Dom know you're enjoying yourself (or if a limit is being reached). Understanding that you aren't "ruining" a scene by needing to stop and say, "Actually, that isn't working for me" is not a bad thing; it's the opposite. It shows you know your limits and aren't afraid to speak up for yourself.

If you don't feel like you're ready to communicate openly with a partner throughout a scene, *you're not ready to jump into a scene yet.* Sharpen these skills first. This can look like talking through fantasy together, co-creating safe words and boundaries, and getting really clear about what you want during a scene before the scene starts. Being submissive does not mean you get to just throw up your hands and let everything be "done to you." You're just as involved in the scene as your Dom.

## Attunement

Effective subbing means being in tune with oneself. "A good sub is somebody who is really attuned to their emotional capabilities, their past experiences and traumas, especially things that they know might trigger them or might upset them or harm them," says Reed Amber. "For example, being called certain words or certain names. Some people could love the term 'filthy slut' and other people could really be repulsed by that term."

Attunement also means being in touch with your Dom—and being able to feel out the energy of the scene. Sure, the Dom is going to be doling out the spankings, but the scene is about connection as much as it is about power exchange.

## Flexibility and willingness to explore

A good sub understands that experiences will be different with different Doms—and therefore, things you try with one person might not work for you, but that doesn't necessarily mean they won't work with someone else.

Now, I'm not suggesting that you should try something you're not into or did not enjoy at all, but oftentimes we aren't totally sure if something is for us right away. Having an openness to trying an act, a dynamic, or a scene more than once can be a good learning experience.

For example, if you were with a partner in the past who wanted to do spanking and you didn't enjoy that experience, you might want to give it another go with a new partner. Everyone is different and will offer something different when it comes to spanking.

Or maybe you tried bondage with your partner and got triggered during that experience. Perhaps it gave you some anxiety. After some reassurance and a plan for if that were to happen again (hello, safe words!), you decide to give it another go. Knowing you can trust your partner and having new knowledge about what to expect could lead to you feeling differently about it.

It's really about a willingness to be flexible and open to new experiences. Amber Reed says that when you really trust your Dom, you can start to allow them to push your boundaries a little bit, to see how far they can take you in certain play to experience more pleasure or sensation. This won't be for everyone, but it can work for some D/s relationships. When we're super rigid in our play, we can limit ourselves.

With that being said, flexibility isn't for everyone. If being specific and contained is what you want, more power to you. Again, there is no wrong or right way to engage in D/s dynamics and play. For some neurodivergent folx, for example, they might find a lot of release and comfort in having a very specific scene, where very specific actions are played out, in a very specific order. They might be very content and happy with this arrangement, and have no desire to stray from the status quo. There's nothing wrong with this. Different strokes for different folx. It's all about getting what you want from the scene to feel like your authentic sub self.

**AGONY AUNT QUESTION AND ANSWER: I want to be a sub, but I'm afraid to give up control**

Q *Dear Auntie Gigi,*

*I've always wanted to be a submissive during sex, but I've never permitted myself to do so. I'm trans masc and have always been expected to be the more dominant one in the bedroom. Or, at the very least, it feels that way. I mostly date AFAB people and femmes. Honestly, it feels like I'm performing masculinity sometimes, and I'm not down for that.*

*What I really am is a submissive person who is curious about bondage. I want my partner to take control and tie me up. But, here's the big thing: I'm really scared to give up control. I have a history of sexual assault in the past, and I find the vulnerability necessary to ask for what I want—and then to do it—super intimidating. What if I freak out and hate it? It's a lot. So, what do I do? How do I feel safe giving up control? And how do I ask my partner to even try this with me? Help!*

*Sub Under the Surface*

Dear Sub Under the Surface,

A There are so many interwoven layers to this narrative. You feel like you're performing masculinity with partners, you're conflicted about embracing your submissive side, and you feel you're expected to be dominant with your partner, whether true or imagined. So, first, don't guilt yourself for finding all of this difficult. A lot is going on here, and being gentle with yourself is important.

OK, first, let's talk about how to get your partner on board with being more dominant. Then, we can dive into how to feel safe giving up control. Here are some ways to make it happen.

**Have conversation(s) outside of the bedroom**

The first conversations to have should center on sexual expectations—namely, why you believe you are expected to be dominant during sex. Getting a clearer understanding of what you perceive to be expected of you and what is actually expected of you could be quite eye-opening. You might find out that this is something you've created, and reality reflects something different. Then again, maybe not. Either way, roles can shift. Getting into the weeds about expectations and what you do and do not want will open you up for deeper conversations about the roles you want to explore that might not fit into typical masculine stereotypes. Who even has time for trying to smash themselves into a gender box, right?

If you want your partner to get into some domination,

don't expect them to suddenly be a rope Top out of nowhere. These types of fantasies and scenes need to be talked about beforehand, outside of the bedroom.

This can get a little awkward, but if you're in a trusting and healthy relationship, there's no reason why you can't have these types of talks. Allow your partner to voice their concerns and desires, too. If this is an out-of-character way you'd like them to behave, they may be a bit apprehensive. Make space for apprehension and come to the conversation with empathy—from both sides!

Co-collaborate around the scene. You say you're a submissive who wants to try bondage. Well, what kind of submissive? Do you see yourself being totally sub or more of a brat? What kind of bondage are we talking about here? Rope? Cage? Handcuffs? Get clear here.

Remember that this is a sexual adventure for the two of you together. It's an experience you're sharing.

### Explore some erotic material that is in line with your fantasies

If your partner is down to explore, but you don't really know where to begin, watch some bondage porn together—from queer-friendly sites like PinkLabel.TV and Erika Lust. Get some ideas. Obviously, porn is not a representation of real-life sex, but it can certainly act as a turn-on. You can also explore erotica and pornographic books together.

Anything you use to get the steam rising is a good start. Talk about your fantasies, get some inspiration, and enjoy yourselves.

### Boost your partner's ego – and make room for your ego, too

One thing that will really get your partner going and into this new, dominant role is boosting their ego. Make it a point to tell them how hot you find it when they take charge. And those affirmations can go both ways. If your partner can let you know how much they enjoy seeing you submit, you'll feel more confident getting into your role.

This, too, can feel a bit awkward at first, but if you want to really make this dynamic happen, you've got to be willing to get your partner and yourself into the right headspace.

Alright, let's talk about the fear of letting go. You're not alone in this. The desire to be submissive and being scared shitless of actually being submissive can exist at the same time. It's a very vulnerable position to be submissive, and it takes trust in both your Dom and yourself.

I want to acknowledge and validate how difficult it can be to want to explore your submissive side while also healing from sexual assault. This is no easy feat, but it doesn't have to limit you from embracing your submissive self. It only means you have to approach it with more intentionality and care than you otherwise would. Start by thinking through your triggers. What about bondage makes you feel uneasy? What kinds of emotions does it bring up for you? Getting clear here can be a big step forward. I would recommend three things to consider:

*Get clear on your boundaries and safe words.*

You want to have a container set up in a way that feels as

safe as possible. If you're going to hand control over to your partner, this doesn't mean you have no control over what happens to you. You are entitled to have your boundaries respected. So, clearly articulate safe words (or safe gestures) that can help you feel safer. And have a post-play plan in place. Consider what would make you feel safe and contained post-scene. Is it cuddling? Talking things through? Maybe being wrapped up in a blanket like a little kitten?

*Try the lightest of light bondage first.*

We often think that we need to jump right into master-level Shibari if we want to try bondage. And don't get me wrong, Shibari can be so much fun. But if you're new to bondage and aren't sure how you're going to respond to it, I'd suggest keeping things light and simple. A low-key pair of trick handcuffs can be amazing because they're easy to remove. Bondage and submission don't mean immediately throwing all caution to the wind. Baby steps and taking things slowly can ensure you're moving into your submissive role in a way that feels safe for you.

*Even if it's hard, communicate with your partner.*

You absolutely do not have to give the details of your sexual assault to your partner. This is not the important thing here. What's important is that your partner knows that there *is* a history of some kind and that it could result in your being triggered. It's about building awareness and connection between the two of you so that they can stay attuned to you during a scene. If you don't feel safe sharing this with your partner, I would caution against throwing yourselves into a D/s dynamic, as they won't have the information they need to adequately keep you safe. And honestly, we shouldn't be playing with Doms we don't trust anyway.

And, because this cannot be overstated, go slowly and have compassion for yourself. You very well may become triggered, and that is OK—you just have to have a plan in place to make sure you can feel safe and secure as quickly as possible. The more you can practice trust and containment, the easier the play will become. You're not weird for craving the freedom of submission while being worried about letting go. This is something you can work with, as long as you're taking care and being intentional.

Now, although you seem very sure that you're a sub and I love that for you, remember that it is also OK to decide you don't like being submissive—or that you *do*, but bondage actually isn't your thing. It's all about being flexible, open to experience, and learning about yourself. We have to give ourselves the space we need to try different kinds of play to determine what feels authentic for us.

I hope this helps you on your journey, little sub! I'm so happy for you and this big, exciting adventure.

XOXO Auntie Gigi

## WHAT ABOUT "SWITCHES"?

You don't have to choose between being a Dom or being a sub. There is so much delicious nuance in kink. You may find that you're a Dom in some relationships, contexts, scenes, or with certain partners—but you're a massive, horny little sub in other circumstances. You just might be a switch.

What's more, you don't have to be 50/50 split between a Dom or sub. You may have a preference for one role over the other—and then again, maybe not. Every single person is different, and the ways their switchiness plays out will depend on what feels right for them in the moment, on the day, or in the scene. You might even find that you want to switch mid-scene—and that's completely OK as long as everyone involved is on board.

You might identify as:

* Top/switch
* bottom/switch

* Dom/switch
* sub/switch.

You may rarely engage in your other role, but you're still a switch, babe.

And if you're not sure if you're a switch yet, that's also—you guessed it—OK! Self-discovery is a process. Take gay men figuring out if they're vers, for example. A survey from *The Archives of Sexual Behavior* found that when it came to figuring out labels for participants, "men's sexual position self-label was learned over a 15-year timespan." Know you're not alone when it comes to being unsure about which label works for you, or what kind of sexual role you want to play. Essentially, most of us are still figuring it out.

Ty David Lerman, a psychotherapist and certified sex thera-pist, told me in an interview that what's needed is a willingness to learn about yourself. "The most important part of this is to adopt a curious mindset," he says. "Get curious about your fantasies, your literal dreams, to what you're attracted to." These can help guide you along the path to figuring out what you like and how you identify.

## HOW TO TELL IF "SWITCH" IS YOUR BAG

To figure out if this label vibes with you, accredited psychosexual and relationship psychotherapist Silva Neves tells me that experimentation with different roles can be very useful. "It is important to go slow with the experiments, and preferably with someone that is trustworthy and patient," he says.

Neves says that labels or sexual preferences are often context-dependent, too. Meaning, you may be exclusively interested in Topping with one partner, down to bottom with another, and very open to switching with another.

Your label preferences may also change with time and experience. You may go through periods of your life where you only want to Top or only want to bottom. Or you may find you're into being a sub at one point and a Domtastic Dom at another. This is valid.

Last, you don't even have to choose a label at all if you don't want to. "Some people don't want to label themselves because they believe that having sex with [someone] is much more than a position preference and such labels are reductive," Neves says.

## WHO AM I TODAY? DOM? TOP? SUB? BOTTOM?

We've already broken down in Chapter 2 what a Dom, sub, Top, and bottom are in terms of power dynamics. There are key differences between Domming and Topping, and between subbing and bottoming, and these are very relevant when we're talking about a switchy dynamic, because not every scene is going to be strictly D/s.

You may be a switch who enjoys being in control, or giving up control in a particular dynamic or context, but you don't want that control to fall into a Dominant/submissive dynamic. You want things done to you (or to do the things), but without the D/s part.

For example, it's very possible to want to spank your partner with a flogger, but not want the action to be entirely capital D Dominant. You may be feeling like you're in more of a Top energy moment. You want to give the spanking, but you want the dynamic to be more about the giving and receiving of sensation, rather than the D/s vibes. This is a perfectly valid way to engage with kink.

Intimacy coordinator Rufai Ajala (Roo) says that in their experience, Dom and sub are more linked to actual identities that people feel quite deeply to their cores, while Top and bottom are more about the contexts and actions of the scenes. Of course, some folx may very well consider their Top/bottom roles to be a part of their identity. It's all entirely subjective.

When deciding what kind of role you're feeling at any given time, ask yourself these five essential questions:

* What kind of energy do I have right now, at this moment? Am I feeling like I'm in a Top mood? A Dom mood? A sub mood? Or do I want to bottom?

* What kind of vibe do I want this scene/act to have? What dynamic am I looking to create?

* What is my partner's role in this scene—what do they want in this context?

- Where do powerplay dynamics come in, in this particular context? How do I want my power exchange to manifest right now?

- What kind of outcome am I hoping to garner from this scene? How do I want to leave feeling?

Unpicking where you are at any given moment, and in any given context, can help you figure out where your head is and what you're feeling. It's important to have open and honest conversations with your partner about what kind of role you're currently aligning with, to temper and align expectations.

Here are five examples of effectively communicating if you're in your Top/bottom/Dom/sub energy.

- I'm really feeling like I'm in my Dom energy today. Would you be open to playing with that in mind?

- I'm in a sub mindset today. I would love to experience [insert what kind of scene and/or dynamic you're picturing]. Are you open to being Dom?

- Where is your head today? I've had a really long week, but I'd love to play. I'm in my Top energy today, not so much Dom. Would you be down to do [insert kink activity]?

- I'm feeling very bottom. To me, that means [insert what bottoming means to you in this context]. Are you down for that?

- I'm frothing at the mouth to be Dom right now. How do you feel about that?

**AGONY AUNT QUESTION AND ANSWER:** I'm a switch, but my partner is fully submissive. What should I do?

Q*Dear Auntie Gigi,*

*I've (28F) been with my partner (29F) for nearly three years now. We've had a pretty good relationship, with a lot of fun and healthy kink play involved. For the most part, I consider myself a Dom. It's where I've had the majority of my experience, both in this relationship and before it. And I do love it! I'm very comfortable in my Mistress role.*

*While I am a Dom, I really am a switch underneath it all. I've found that there are so few Tops in the kink world, and we're in such high demand that I've had little opportunity to ever explore my submissive side. Everyone is looking for a Dom, you know? As time has gone on, the desire to explore my subby nature has increased more and more. I want to embrace it and engage in play that can facilitate this.*

*Here's the problem: My partner is 100 percent sub right down to her sweet little bones. She's a very gentle type. She likes being tied up, beaten in the most delicious ways, and told she's a perfect, good girl for taking it all. It's all quite wholesome.*

*I'm not sure what to do here. Can I explore my submissive side in a way that doesn't compromise my relationship or my partner's desires? I don't want to make her do anything she doesn't want to do, but at the same time, I feel like I'm compromising my own needs as a result. Do I bring this up with her? Or should I just suck it up and deal? Any advice?*

*Switch Dom*

Dear Switch Dom,

First, I'm just gushing over your description of your relationship. It really does sound so lovely and wholesome in the kinkiest way. And I love that for you! I'm always so happy when a couple can explore and play in the taboo in a way that feels safe and fulfilling.

With that being said, there is absolutely nothing wrong with wanting to explore your submissive side. Human beings are nothing if not complex, and having desires across the spectrum is completely normal and healthy.

I totally hear you about the abundance of subs and the widespread need for Doms. This seems to be an ongoing community dilemma, but such is life, eh? A sea full of bottoms and not a Top in sight! What a world.

I certainly don't think you should just "suck it up and deal." This feels like a one-way ticket to Resentment Town—both for your kink practice and for your partner. Sure, it's not your partner's fault that she's a subby sub and might not have any interest in Domming, but that doesn't make her needs any more important than yours.

The first thing that needs to happen is sussing out what kind of submissive role you're interested in. Do you see yourself in the same submissive, masochistic, good girl role as your partner? Maybe your fantasy is very different, and so is the *kind* of submissive you want to be. Also, consider the acts you're interested in. Since you haven't had a whole lot of first-hand sub experience, it might be helpful to think this through based on your limited sub experience and the feedback you've received from both your girlfriend and other partners.

Last, how do you see this manifesting? Is it a one-time thing? An ongoing or occasional dynamic? Or would you want to move into subbing as a full-time thing? Reflect on all of this as much as possible until you have a clear idea of what you want. This will help you communicate your needs much more easily.

Next, and this is the hard part, it's time to sit down and have an open and honest discussion with your partner. She might be totally on board with exploring this with you, and that would be super great! But it's not a guarantee—and while I can't make assumptions, based on your description, it is very possible she won't want to take on the Dom role you're craving. Be prepared to accept a "No, thank you" with kindness and empathy.

But do not think this is the end of the road! Just because your partner isn't interested doesn't mean you have to cut off your submissive desires.

Based on your letter, I'm going to assume you and your partner are currently monogamous—but this next advice is applicable regardless of your relationship structure. Your partner's reluctance could be a beautiful opportunity to discuss and collaborate on ways you can have these needs met elsewhere. Perhaps there is a professional Dom you could hire to session with you. Or you could find a BDSM sex party in your neighborhood or in the closest city, where you could attend alone or with your partner. You could even try a kink-friendly dating app and find kink play partners that way, explicitly stating that you're looking for a play partner only. It's not our partner's obligation to be the one to fill every single sexual, kinky, or erotic need—but if they don't want to, they should be open to figuring out a solution that works for both of you. It's all about communication, setting boundaries that work for both of you, and having ongoing check-ins to ensure everyone is feeling safe, happy, and content.

Your needs are valid and deserve to be explored if they are important to you. The road may be a bit rough and rocky, but you can get there. It might be helpful to get a kink-informed, LGBTQ+-friendly sex therapist to act as a mediator for these conversations. Having another party there to help navigate these fraught conversations can be extremely useful.

I hope this helps you on your journey, and you get everything you want and more.

XOXO Auntie Gigi

Hopefully, by now, as we close this chapter, you're starting to feel more assured and secure in the role you want to play in BDSM, whether that be Dom, sub, or switch. Our kink identities are such an integral part of intentional play, and the more we dare to explore the meaning we find in them, the deeper we can get into our kink practice.

Remember that it takes self-compassion, empathy, and a whole lot of patience to get fully comfortable within our kink identities, and that they may shift and change over time. Be gentle with yourself. You've got this.

## Chapter 10 recap

In Chapter 10, we bravely began exploring different roles in kink dynamics and how you can start to embrace your kink identity most effectively for yourself and your journey. We laid out the kink spectrum and how we might find ourselves falling somewhere on the gradient, rather than into black and white roles, because, you know, humans are complex.

We broke down the ways to be your most authentic (and intentional) Dom or sub. We then explored thematic reader questions to gain more perspective on each of these roles.

Last, we took a look at switches and their place in the BDSM world. We explored how to know if you're in Top/bottom or Dom/sub energy and looked at a few examples of how to communicate this mindset to someone you're playing with.

## JOURNAL PROMPTS

1.  For the Doms: Why do I want to be a Dom? What about it is appealing to me? What do I want to get out of this role and experience?

2.  For the subs: Why do I want to be a sub? What about it is appealing to me? What do I want to get out of this role and experience?

3.  For the Doms: What kind of Dom do I want to be? What kind of character and scene(s) am I envisioning?

4.  For the subs: What kind of sub do I want to be? What kind of character and scene(s) am I envisioning?

5.  For the Doms: Consider your emotional needs. What would you need from a scene to feel like your truest Dom self? What would you need from your sub? Reflect.

6.  For the subs: Consider your emotional needs. What would you need from a scene to feel like your truest submissive self? What would you need from your Dom to feel safe, contained, and seen? Reflect.

7.  Switches: Consider your last sexual encounter. What kind of energy were you in? What was the context? Consider how you were feeling, the environment, the partner you were with, and so forth. Starting to pick apart what triggers your inner Dom/sub/Top/bottom can be essential for understanding yourself better in the moment and before constructing scenes.

8.  For Doms, subs, and switches: What do I want to feel during a scene? How do I want to be treated during the scene by my partner?

## EXERCISES

**EXERCISE 1:** Conditions for good kink

This exercise is modified from the source material "Conditions for Good Sex" that appears in *Mind the Gap* by Dr. Karen Gurney (2020).

The conditions for good kink are very similar to the conditions that make for good sex, only they include kink-specific themes like sensation and safety, though both of these things are important in both kink and sex in general.

The Conditions for Good Kink Triangle

1.   Physical touch and sensations

2.   Psychological arousal

3.   Safety and presence

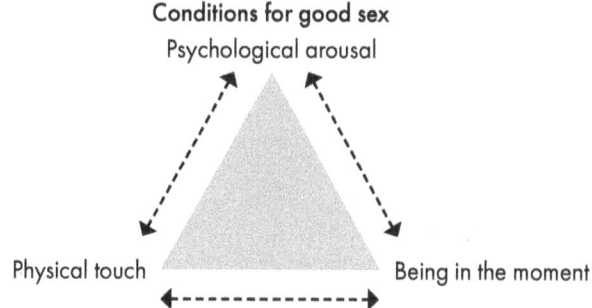

**Conditions for good sex**
Psychological arousal

Physical touch                    Being in the moment

Physical touch and sensation refer to the actions within the scene. This includes the types of play, toys, equipment, outfits, and punishments that are included in the scene. These physical sensations need to be in line with your preferences to have a good, consensual kink experience.

Psychological arousal refers to all the things that get you going in that big, beautiful brain of yours. This includes the power dynamics being explored, the roles each partner is adopting, the kinds of dirty talk and language being used, and the environment you're in.

Safety and presence may seem like two different things, but they are intertwined in kink. Safety is essential for presence. Good kink happens when we're able to let go into our roles safely, feeling secure and confident that our limits and boundaries will be respected.

Draw your own triangle and get ready to write. For each of the conditions for good kink, write your own. These should be as close to your ideal scenario as possible. Take some time to think about this and reflect.

## EXERCISE 2: The themes of kink

Identifying common themes can be a really useful way to start unpacking what it is you want out of kink. If you haven't explored kink before in any context, you're free to use any past sexual experiences to draw from.

1.  Situation/scene/sexual experience

    . . . . . . . . . . . . . . . . . . . . . . . . . . . . . . . . . . . . . . . . . . . . . . . . . .

    a.  Good things about this experience

        . . . . . . . . . . . . . . . . . . . . . . . . . . . . . . . . . . . . . . . . . . . . . . . .

    b.  Bad or unfavorable things about this experience

        . . . . . . . . . . . . . . . . . . . . . . . . . . . . . . . . . . . . . . . . . . . . . . . .

2.  Situation/scene/sexual experience

    . . . . . . . . . . . . . . . . . . . . . . . . . . . . . . . . . . . . . . . . . . . . . . . . . . .

    a.  Good things about this experience

        . . . . . . . . . . . . . . . . . . . . . . . . . . . . . . . . . . . . . . . . . . . . . . . .

    b.  Bad or unfavorable things about this experience

        . . . . . . . . . . . . . . . . . . . . . . . . . . . . . . . . . . . . . . . . . . . . . . . .

3.  Situation/scene/sexual experience

    . . . . . . . . . . . . . . . . . . . . . . . . . . . . . . . . . . . . . . . . . . . . . . . . . . .

    a.  Good things about this experience

        . . . . . . . . . . . . . . . . . . . . . . . . . . . . . . . . . . . . . . . . . . . . . . . .

    b.  Bad or unfavorable things about this experience

        . . . . . . . . . . . . . . . . . . . . . . . . . . . . . . . . . . . . . . . . . . . . . . . .

Common good themes

. . . . . . . . . . . . . . . . . . . . . . . . . . . . . . . . . . . . . . . . . . . . .

Common bad themes

. . . . . . . . . . . . . . . . . . . . . . . . . . . . . . . . . . . . . . . . . . . . .

What I learned from this exercise

. . . . . . . . . . . . . . . . . . . . . . . . . . . . . . . . . . . . . . . . . . . . .

## EXERCISE 3: The BDSM test

How to figure out if you're a Dom or sub? Take the BDSM quiz! Go to: https://bdsmtest.org/select-mode. This quiz can help you figure out where your kinks lie and what seems to be most important to you. It offers helpful percentage breakdowns to help you decode what kinds of kinks and play are most important to you.

## EXERCISE 4: Worksheet—Your limits and boundaries

Fill out the following sections to the best of your ability in short answer form.

1. What does kink mean to me? Is it a fun thing to try during sex, a lifestyle, a way of connecting with my partner, a 24/7 dynamic?

2. My role during kink is _____ (Dom, sub, switch), and I want that role to manifest as...(Mommy/Daddy, pet/Pet Owner, slave/Master).

3. I enjoy kink play because _____ (power dynamics, having

fun, trying something new, desire to please my partner, experiencing different sensations, etc.).

4. During a kink scene, I want to feel _____.

5. I am hoping to get _____ out of this scene.

6. My main concerns about engaging in this play are _____.

# 11

## AM I BROKEN?

### How to Embrace Your Kinks and Fetishes in an Authentic Way

---

**What you'll find in this chapter:**

→ Purity culture, shame, and how these impact our sexuality.

→ Authentic integration and the power of fantasy.

- How to map out fantasies and decide what should stay in the fantasy realm and what you want to make in real life.

→ Agony Aunt question and answer.

→ Exercises.

---

**L**et's get real for a second. You cannot fully embrace your authentic, kinky self without first looking shame dead in the eye. And you can't understand that shame without unpacking the heavy weight of purity culture.

So let's start there, because this is where so much of our inner conflict begins.

If you've ever had a moment where your desires made you feel guilty, weird, dirty, broken, or "too much," you're not alone. That shame didn't come from nowhere. It was put there. Often subtly. Sometimes overtly. But always powerfully. And here's the truth: It's not your fault.

The messages of shame around sexuality—especially around desire, fantasy, kink, and anything non-normative—are woven into the very fabric of our culture. Even if you weren't raised in a religious home, even if your parents were liberal or atheist, you've likely still been exposed to purity culture in one form or another. It's that pervasive.

Just look at the kind of sex education most of us received growing up in Western societies: abstinence-first, fear-based, shame-soaked. Sex is framed as something inherently dangerous, dirty, or taboo—something that must be controlled, restricted, or repressed. That entire framework? That's purity culture.

And it goes further. Consider the spiritual messaging that tells people to "cleanse" their genitals with sage or ritual baths to rid themselves of the energy of past lovers, as if our bodies are dirty by default and need to be purified after pleasure. Or the way kink is pathologized—dismissed as a sign of trauma, dysfunction, or moral failing.

None of this is by accident. Purity culture has shaped the way we talk about sex, the way we teach about sex, and the way we feel about sex.

And that shame? It's not just intellectual. It lives in the body. Whether you've freshly thrown off the shackles of purity culture, are attempting to do so presently, or escaped a long time ago, let's break down how purity culture impacts sexuality and how you can start to unlearn these messages to embrace pleasure, kink, and sexual freedom to the fullest extent.

## WHAT IS PURITY CULTURE?

At its most basic definition, purity culture is a belief system that centers sexuality around morality, with "purity" defined by the absence of sexual experience, especially for women and those raised female.

It teaches that your worth, value, goodness, and even your spiritual integrity are directly tied to your sexual behavior. In most forms, this means abstaining from any kind of sexual activity until marriage. But in practice, it goes way deeper.

As Dr. Laurie Mintz, psychologist and author of *Becoming Cliterate*, shared with me, purity culture isn't just about abstinence. It's about control, especially control of female sexuality.

Within many fundamentalist frameworks—particularly Evangelical Christianity—girls and women are taught that not only should they abstain from sex, but they also bear responsibility for men's thoughts, urges, and behaviors. They are instructed to dress modestly, act passively, and always avoid "tempting" the men around them. They are expected to be gatekeepers of male sexuality while being utterly disconnected from their own.

In this system, a woman's value lies in her submission, her modesty, and her ability to suppress her own pleasure for the sake of others. And while purity culture targets everyone to some extent, it disproportionately affects women, femmes, queer people, trans folx, and anyone whose sexuality falls outside of cis-heteronormative ideals.

## WHAT PURITY CULTURE MESSAGING LOOKS LIKE IN REAL LIFE

Even if we never set foot in a church or sat through an abstinence lecture, these ideas are in the air we breathe. They're echoed in pop culture, relationships, education systems, and media. Sometimes they slip into our minds in quiet, insidious ways. Here are just a few examples:

*   comparing sexually active women to "chewed-up gum" that no one would want

*   being told that if you have sex before marriage, you're "used up" or "damaged goods"

*   blaming women and girls for men's behavior ("You must've tempted him")

*   teaching that a "good" woman is always submissive

*   equating spiritual worth with sexual abstinence and suppression

*   claiming that watching porn = addiction = hell

*   shaming anyone with non-vanilla desires

*   saying kink is a result of trauma and therefore proof that you're sick or broken.

## THE LINGERING IMPACT OF SHAME ON SEXUALITY

Shame is not just a feeling—it's an emotional state that tells you that you are fundamentally wrong, bad, or broken. And when shame gets wrapped around your sexuality, it creates a deep disconnection between your mind and body.

Even when we consciously reject purity culture later in life, the residue of shame lingers. You might try to embrace your desires, but find yourself feeling guilty afterwards. You might fantasize about kink, but feel like something is wrong with you for doing so. You might crave connection, but struggle to feel safe in your body.

That's because your mind and body need to feel safe to feel desire and arousal, and to experience orgasm. When shame or fear is activated, the body can go into a state of fight, flight, or freeze, which cuts off access to pleasure. It creates internal conflict, tension, and emotional distance.

Instead of relaxing into your sexuality, you may find yourself dissociating, shutting down, or spiraling into critical self-talk.

Here are some examples of how the trauma of purity culture messaging can lead to sexual difficulties:

- feeling emotionally or physically numb during sex
- believing that sexual difficulties are your fault
- avoiding conversations about sex altogether
- pain during sex or sexual performance struggles
- rushing through intimacy or needing substances to engage
- feeling like you're "too much" or "not enough"

- difficulty experiencing playfulness or spontaneity

- trouble reaching orgasm

- feeling undeserving of pleasure

- staying stuck in unfulfilling sexual patterns

- deep shame around your kinks—even after exploring them.

And, of course, feeling a shitload of shame around having kinky desires—which may lead to you not wanting to explore them, trying to suppress them, or engaging with them and feeling like crap afterwards. It's not good, is what I'm saying.

## SIX WAYS TO HEAL FROM PURITY CULTURE AND RECLAIM YOUR KINK

If you're a purity culture dropout (honestly, most of us are in some way), here's how you can start reclaiming your sexuality and embracing your kink—shame-free.

### 1. Give yourself time to heal

Escaping purity culture is no small feat. But healing takes time, space, and compassion. As Rowett says, "Remember to give yourself a lot of time and space to heal, and know that you don't need to figure it all out now." You've been carrying these messages for years—be gentle with yourself as you begin to release them. Plus, I have some fun and reliable exercises for you that can help you let go of shame in your own time. I'm proud of you!

## 2. Feel your damn feelings

This work can bring up sadness, grief, anger, and frustration. Let it. "You might feel sad and want to mourn the lost years of your sex life," Phillips explains. "You might feel angry, or personally victimized. You may feel hurt. Whatever is there to feel, feel it fully."

## 3. Find your people

Start with books, podcasts, or documentaries like *Pure* or *Deconstructing My Religion*. Join online forums or communities where others are deconstructing purity culture, too. Better yet, explore kink-friendly spaces and apps like Feeld—not just for dating, but for finding like-minded community.

## 4. Work with a professional

"Unlearning such toxic, harmful messages is difficult—but with education and support, it is possible," Mitz says. Find a sex therapist, coach, or support group that specifically works with purity culture survivors. There's real power in being witnessed and supported by someone who understands the nuances of this healing work. Rowett even has amazing classes that are centered on embracing your pleasure and leaving shame in the past. You should Google her!

## 5. Practice conscious masturbation

This is about more than getting off—it's about reconnecting with your body. Try slowing down, breathing deeply, and being fully present in your pleasure. Even just practicing soft touch with no goal can help you feel safer in your skin. It is a brilliant way to come into yourself and embrace that your body is a vessel for pleasure. And that you deserve pleasure!

### 6. Practice conscious kink

That's what this whole book is about. But beyond technique, this is about staying connected to your body and pleasure in a way that is intentional, healing, and empowering. If you need guidance, check out the conscious kink exercises in the next section—you can even try them solo.

## AUTHENTIC INTEGRATION AND THE POWER OF FANTASY

A huge component of letting go of shame around our desires is figuring out how we want to authentically integrate them into our lives. This can be in real-life play or fantasy. The latter is incredibly important to integration in kink. Fantasy is the foundational layer that allows us to play with our desires in a safe, non-intimidating way.

So, let's talk about fantasy and the ways we can engage with it to release shame and feel grounded in our kinkiest of kinky desires.

## LET'S NOT GET IT TWISTED: YOUR FANTASY ISN'T "CREEPY" OR "WEIRD"

First of all, we need to chill out about having sexual fantasies. Fantasies aren't weird, gross, creepy, or horrible. They don't make you a bad person, no matter the fantasy you're having. And everyone is having one kind of fantasy or another.

Our minds are astoundingly complex. They can come up with

some of the most fantastical things you've ever imagined. The brain is our most powerful sex organ, and it can control much more than we realize. You know how you can convince yourself that someone is breaking into your house to murder you in the night based on a noise you heard outside your room? This is not steeped in reality, and yet your brain has convinced you it is plausible. Don't underestimate the power of your thoughts.

When it comes to thoughts of sex and kink, everything is really "normal." Sure, some sexual acts aren't acceptable in real life such as rape, necrophilia, and so forth. Anything that doesn't involve explicit consent from everyone involved should never be acted upon.

However, even if you have a fantasy that falls into one of these "dark" or "disturbing" categories, you aren't insane or mentally ill. According to Dr. Justin Lehmiller's survey of over 4000 people, many people have fantasies like this (think necrophilia and non-consensual voyeurism). We can concoct some wild things up in our noggins.

Of course, there are some cases where there may be a need to take action. If you're having repeated or persistent fantasies of a disturbing nature that you can't seem to control, that's when you should probably seek therapy. Otherwise, stop beating yourself up. People are bizarre, and you are by no means the only one thinking about weird stuff.

## FANTASIES AREN'T ALWAYS BASED ON REAL-LIFE PREFERENCES

Keep in mind that just because you think about a certain kinky situation, it doesn't mean you necessarily want to act on it. Many of us have sexual ideas or fantasies that turn us on that would not be hot to try in real life. For instance, perhaps you think a lot about getting pissed on, but you know that if you got pissed on in real life, it would be more gross to you than hot. It might turn you on in thought, but in practice, it just wouldn't work for you.

This is completely legitimate. You can have a kink for water sports without actually wanting to do water sports.

Not every fantasy is a reflection of real-life preferences. You might watch a bunch of intense bondage porn, but the idea of being tied up in real life doesn't appeal to you. When working to authentically integrate your kinks in a way that feels right for you, it's crucial to distinguish whether or not this is something you'd like to act upon or if it's just something that gets you going in thought.

## FIVE STEPS TO MAP OUT FANTASIES AND DECIDE WHAT SHOULD STAY IN THE FANTASY REALM AND WHAT YOU WANT TO MAKE IN REAL LIFE

### Step 1: Choose your fantasy of focus

We rarely have only one fantasy, so getting specific with a scene of focus can be useful. Think about the thing that sparks your *peak* sexual excitement. What happens in the scene where you feel this excitement? Think through the fantasy from start to finish. Try to imagine as much detail as possible.

### Step 2: Allow your fantasy to take on the edge of real life

OK, so now let's try to think about what this would look like in practice. Who might be there? What thoughts might come up for you? Is this something that could be done safely? Consider how you might feel if you were able to live this fantasy out and ask yourself: Would I want that?

### Step 3: Try it out alone

Obviously, a lot of fantasies involve other people, but you can begin to straddle the fantasy and in-real-life realm by doing as much of the scene as you can on your own. For instance, if you're picturing a gang bang scene, get on the bed and use a bunch of different toys to simulate the gang bang scene. Use your imagination to bring the other people into the room. Ask yourself again: Would I want that?

### Step 4: Make the leap (or don't)

Decide where this fantasy lives. Maybe you've walked through all of these steps so far and have decided this one's rooted firmly in Imagination Land. Maybe you've decided you want to try it in real life, or would be open to it in the right context. Maybe you're in one camp with the notion that this could change. Whatever it is you decide, that's legit. You can always, always, always change your mind!

### Step 5: Have compassion for yourself, baby!

Have compassion (looooads of it) for yourself when you're looking more closely at your fantasies. You're putting yourself in a risky place, even if that risk is mostly self-perceived. Self-compassion is so crucial when it comes to exploring sexual interests that fall outside society's norms. We have to take in, process, and try to understand the emotions that come up. Sometimes these emotions can be very uncomfortable or difficult. Be brave enough to sit with those uncomfortable feelings.

Being able to be vulnerable with yourself about your desires shows a lot of strength. Be gentle with yourself, because you deserve gentleness, you wonderful little pervert.

**AGONY AUNT QUESTION AND ANSWER: I fantasize about being spanked, but when I orgasm, I feel so ashamed afterwards. What is going on?**

Q *Dear Auntie Gigi,*

*I should probably start by saying that I do know the source of this shame I'm feeling: I grew up Catholic. My parents were and are still very devout. In the past, I've suffered from pain during sex, which, after a lot of therapy, I figured out was because of this deep-rooted shame I've had around sex. It caused vaginismus. I've done a lot of work to get through this and have made good progress. There is still pain sometimes, but I'm mostly OK.*

*But that isn't why I'm writing to you, Auntie. I have a kink that is causing me serious mental health issues. In my heart of hearts, I want to be spanked. I've never asked anyone to do this before. I can't even imagine doing that. I do, however, masturbate thinking about it all the time. Logically (and from reading your work over the years), I know this is an OK thing to think about. But whenever I orgasm thinking about getting spanked, I feel the most overwhelming and intense shame. It is giving me so much anxiety, to the point where I feel like I might not even want to think about the fantasy anymore. But I really, really don't want to limit myself, and I really enjoy this fantasy. What is going on? Help!*

*Spank Me, I'm Catholic*

A Dear Spank Me, I'm Catholic,

Thank you for your thoughtful question. I'm sorry this is causing you so much distress.

Maybe we should start by considering why this turns you on so much. I wonder if, perhaps, this fantasy is rooted in the often corporal punishment that comes with Catholicism. Two examples come to mind:

1. self-flagellation as a means of repentance

2. the way nuns often smacked the hands of disobedient school children up until the 90s.

Psychologist Evan Sprankle often jokes online that telling someone you grew up Catholic is code for "I'm kinky." I say this to help you get to the root of your fantasy—and hopefully, *why* it causes so much shame. I would be surprised if the two weren't linked. If you get turned on by spanking because of your Catholic roots, you also become deeply ashamed because of your Catholic roots.

What came first? The fantasy or the shame? Only you can answer that question, dearest reader.

But let's talk about the post-climax shame you're experiencing and why that might be.

When we're super, super turned on, the part of our brain that registers disgust and fear essentially gets switched off. Things that we may register as shameful, gross, scary, or weird when we're in a resting state take on erotic meaning once we're turned on.

This is why people enjoy things like water sports, spitting in each other's mouths, electro play, and, in your case, spanking. In the context of everyday life, spanking might not be appealing to you. You wouldn't want to get spanked by someone in a grocery store, for instance. The majority of people require their minds and bodies to be in a sexually aroused state for these more taboo things to be a source of turn-on.

And, believe it or not, it's normal to be aroused by something we'd otherwise find horrifying because of the complex nature of arousal itself. Basically, it boils down to the fact that our brains just aren't that great at figuring out why they're aroused. They just are.

While I can't diagnose you, my psychotherapeutic opinion is that you may be experiencing the post-orgasmic blues, which are amplified to an astronomical degree by shame-related religious trauma. You might be familiar with the colloquial concept of the "afterglow of sex." This is when you feel super great after you orgasm or have sex with someone, or, you know, get spanked. This happens because our bodies are awash with a chemical cocktail of feel-good hormones like dopamine and oxytocin.

But in understanding your dilemma, we have to look at the counterstate: the post-orgasmic (or post-coital) blues (also known as post-coital dysphoria). This denotes the crash that can take place immediately following orgasm.

Sometimes shame can follow orgasm. It happens! The release of all that orgasmic energy doesn't always make us feel amazing in the minutes after sex, especially if we've experienced religious trauma. In fact, the release of that energy can make us feel depleted, sad, lonely, or ashamed of ourselves. Feeling shame, in your case, is all due to the release you experience in orgasm and your religious history. It may manifest as all kinds of emotions—it's a release of tension and intense feelings we've been holding inside.

Both the afterglow and the blues are completely normal and temporary. The two seemingly extreme opposite states are a great example of how complicated human sexuality is.

However, in your case, you're experiencing ongoing and intense anxiety because the release of orgasm is triggering your trauma. It's more than just the blues. Since you find yourself unable to move on from the post-coital funk and are anxious for a prolonged period after sex, I would suggest you seek out the professional help of a qualified therapist who can help you work through your religious trauma and how it relates to your kink.

I want to reiterate that you are not bad or wrong for enjoying spanking. With the help of a qualified therapist (and the exercises in this book), you can start to reframe the shame you have around your kink to find truly authentic integration, whether that be permanently in the fantasy realm or real-life sexual experiences.

I hope this helps!

XOXO Auntie Gigi

Phew, I know this chapter was a heavy one, so I hope you're doing absolutely everything you need to take care of yourself. I suggest taking some time to digest the material before moving on to the journal prompts and exercises. We don't need anyone getting too overwhelmed when we're trying to release shame around kink. Go and have a nice cup of tea, a bath, a walk in nature, or have an orgasm—do whatever it is that most brings you a sense of calm and peace.

### Chapter 11 recap

In Chapter 11, we unpacked shame. We walked through the roots of purity culture in our society and how it can impact our sexuality and how we feel about our more taboo sexual proclivities. The long and short of it is it impacts us a lot, and most of it is not good for the old mental health. Luckily, we also explored some ways to release the shackles of purity culture so we can live more grounded, kinky lives, without all the shame.

Then, we explored the role of fantasy and how it can help us integrate our kinks into our lives in an authentic way. We also looked at six tidy steps to map out a fantasy and decide if it should live in the fantasy realm only or join us earthside. Only you get to make that choice about your kinks.

Finally, we answered a letter from a curious reader who is being severely impacted by religious trauma when it comes to her spanking kink, as well as some advice for how she can begin to heal.

## JOURNAL PROMPTS

1. What role does shame play in your kinks? Does it have a place—or, perhaps, did it have a place at one time?

2. What would it be like to be able to experience your kinks and desires without fear of judgment, shame, or anxiety? Take some time to consider this one because it's important.

3. Reflect on a kink fantasy you want to stay in the fantasy realm. Why is this the case?

4. Reflect on a kink fantasy that you want to bring into your real life. Why is this the case? What would that look like for you?

## EXERCISES

**EXERCISE 1:** Visualization—removing "layers" of shame

Disclaimer: This is an exercise used by many therapists in different forms and fashions across many different disciplines. I first learned about this exercise from my previous clinical supervisor, Silva Neves (whom you've met earlier in this book), and have since used it with countless clients. I do not want to claim this is an original exercise, though it has been written in an original format and adapted to fit the themes of this work.

I'm going to walk you through an exercise in which we're going to imagine shame and harmful messages we've received about our kinks and desires as layers of clothing. Before you try this exercise, read it thoroughly. If you prefer, read it out loud on a voice note and then play the voice note back with your eyes closed. I wish I could read it out loud to you, but alas, we are trapped in these pages. Let's begin.

Close your eyes. Take a few deep breaths. Now, imagine you're standing on the edge of a large, rocky cliff. The sky is overcast. The wind is brisk and blowing through your hair. It's so strong it feels like it should be blowing right through you to your bones. But it doesn't. You're very, very warm, buried under layers and layers of garments. You feel so heavy. You feel almost suffocated.

You can hear the waves below crashing against the jagged rocks. They are distinct, but you're so high up on the cliff that they feel distant somehow.

Now, look down at your clothes. Examine each layer. Each layer is inscribed with a negative message you've been given—or given yourself—about your desires. What does the first one say? And the second? The third? The fourth? What about the fifth message? Read each one carefully. They are clothes, but they are an extension of you, of your psyche.

Slowly reach down and peel off the first layer. Hold it in your hands. Read the message. Now, ever so gently, release the garment over the cliff. Allow the breeze to pick it up. It whisks it away across the sea. It gets smaller and smaller as it floats away, leaving you. Now, do it again. And again. And again. Watch as each layer of shame and pain and hurt is hurled away into the sky—into the waves.

When you're finished, look down. Your body is light. It is free. You are free. How do you feel?

## EXERCISE 2: Solo conscious kink

Bring back the box breathing exercise from Chapter 9. It is a foundational practice when you're doing this exercise. If you don't remember how to do it, pop back to the exercise section in Chapter 9 to refresh.

The aim of this exercise is self-focus and staying present, which can help us conquer shame by experiencing our kinks in a safe and contained way.

1.  Consider one of your kinks or fetishes.

2.  Practice it alone. This can be challenging for some kinks, but as we discussed earlier, you can use a hybrid in-real-life/fantasy model.

3.  Practice power dynamics with yourself while engaging with this kink. If you're a sub, you're submitting to a Dom side of yourself. If you're a Dom, you're dominating a submissive side to yourself. Yes, you can really self-tie yourself into Shibari ropes (keep the scissors nearby!) or spank yourself with a wooden spoon. You can dress up like a sissy maid and order yourself around. You can tickle your own feet.

4.  Try to stay completely present, utilizing fantasy and box breathing throughout. Focus on sensations in your body. Take special note of difficult emotions that might come up, like shame and embarrassment. Allow yourself to feel those feelings before gently letting them go.

5.  Bring your attention fully to and focus on feelings of pleasure and arousal. Try to follow them.

6.  Reflect:

    a.  What was this experience like for you?

    b.  Did you get anything out of this exercise?

    c.  How does staying present impact shame?

**EXERCISE 3:** The fantasy vs. in real life pros and cons list

What's better for figuring out where kinks should live than a pros and cons list? Pick out the kink you want to work with. It can be the same kink you've used for Exercises 1 and 2, or be something completely new.

Start by really mapping out the kink. Give it a beginning, middle, and end. Who is there? What implements are used, if any? What is everyone doing? Feel free to do this in any format that works for you. You can think about it, write it down, draw, and so forth.

Now, make a pros and cons list for bringing this fantasy in real life.

PROS

CONS

**EXERCISE 4**: Kink gratitude worksheet

Gratitude is the shame-killer. When we can start to reframe the ways we feel about our taboo desires, we can start to set ourselves free. Focusing on the joy and pleasure that kink brings to our lives can rewire the brain away from shame and toward self-actualization. And so, you're going to start a kink-focused gratitude journal. It's just like your regular gratitude journal, only infinitely kinkier—and therefore so much better!

This is a great exercise to repeat whenever those sticky, bad feelings resurface—because they do sometimes.

Prompts to get you started:

1. I am grateful for my kink because...

2. My kink brings _____ (good thing) _____ into my life.

3. In a perfect world, my kink would be in my life in _____ way.

4. When I'm practicing my kink, I want to feel _____.

5. It is not shameful to have my kinks and fantasies because _____.

# 12

# THE SAFETY CONTAINER

## Consent, Safe Words, Limits, Boundaries

### What you'll find in this chapter:

→ Safe words
  • how they work with consent
  • how to create a safe word and meta safe words
  • safe word action plans.
→ Boundaries and limits
  • setting boundaries
    » explicit vs. implicit boundaries
    » hard limits vs. soft limits.
→ A guide to accountability
  • the six steps to take when something goes wrong.
→ Exercises.

T he idea of safe words, boundaries, and limits should not be foreign to you at this point. We've taken a lot of time to set the stage for getting down and dirty with sexy boundaries. All of kink play is built within boundaries. It hinges on consent, safety, and ethics. Our boundaries, limits, and safe words are designed to keep us grounded and secure. Their importance cannot be overstated.

And here you are, ready to take a closer look at the safety container of kink and to begin to create your own set of kinky rules that will help to make your experience feel safe, secure, and sexy AF. OK, let's go!

## SAFE WORDS

A safe word, as we've talked about quite a bit already, is a word or action that is designed to be a failsafe in kink. When a safe word (or gesture) is called, all play stops immediately. Safe words are a part of consent. They mean "a boundary has been reached and I need to take a break." This word is very helpful when you're feeling overwhelmed, upset, or anxious during sex or play.

When you invoke your safe word, you get a chance to reassess what is happening and even talk about what you're feeling. You can always continue with the sexual play after you've had a moment to think and discuss what you need to go forward. These words are an excellent way to maintain your awareness during sexual play.

To violate or ignore someone's safe word is to violate their consent. While a safe word can often be a deeply non-sexual or even hilarious word, it needs to be taken dead seriously.

These safe words are useful for a variety of reasons. Sometimes, in certain sexual or intimate situations, the word "No" doesn't work. For instance, if you're engaged in a ravishment fantasy or a BDSM scene, saying "No" might be a part of your or your partner's character. Meaning, if you say "No," your partner might not know you mean "*No! Stop!*" This has worrying implications. You want to say "No" when you mean "No," but the play doesn't stop. That's scary!

A safe word dissolves any gray area you might experience in these kinds of scenes. When you use the safe word, there is zero doubt about what you mean. This prevents you from going too far when you're not feeling comfortable or safe.

We do not want to force ourselves to stay in a scene or do a kinky act we're not into just to save someone's ego. This is not good for anyone. Yes, communication is hard, but it is so crucial.

If you push yourself through a sexual or kinky act you're not into because you don't want to hurt someone's feelings, you'll probably end up resentful or even traumatized. If you're getting a spanking from your jacked Daddy Dom and it's crossed over from being fun-painful into painful-painful—and you're *not* into that—if you just keep gritting your teeth through it, that's not going to be a good experience. It might even fuck up spanking for you, and we don't want that. Spanking is great.

This is the case for vanilla sex, too. Safe words can (and should) be a part of all sexual experiences. For example, if you're in doggy style and your partner's thrusts become painful rather than pleasurable, you can use your safe word to say, "I'd like this to stop." It's less emotionally fraught than "I hate this. I'm hurting. Get off me." Make sense?

A safe word is an easy out, no matter what you're doing. Discussing having one with your partner sets up predetermined boundaries. We need boundaries when it comes to sex and kink, no matter how much we trust our partners.

## HOW TO CREATE SAFE WORDS

Every safe word is different. Each couple should pick a safe word that works for them. For some, the word "banana" might work. For another couple, "banana" might be too silly or funny. This couple might use something like "apple tree" or "sailboat." It's totally customizable, and you should feel free to have fun with it!

If you're unsure what word to use, talk about it. Have an honest discussion about what would work for both of you. I put a list of suggestions for you at the end of this section, which I really think illustrates how "random" these words can seem, while holding a lot of meaning for you, specifically. For beginners, I suggest using the "traffic light" method from Chapter 7.

You can also choose "meta safe words." Don't worry. It's not as complicated as it sounds. Having a word that means "I'm getting close to a limit" can be really useful. Because, hey, maybe you're feeling unsure, but you don't want the play to fully stop. An alternative word that can let your partner know you're starting to reach the end of your tolerance can let them know that they need to slow down, take a break, or check in with you.

Remember, practice makes perfect. Like all things sexual, it's about finding your groove. Start with the traffic light system and see how it goes.

## 20 FUN AND WACKY SAFE WORDS TO GET YOU GOING, REVVED UP, AND TURNED ON, BABY!

1. Enterprise

2. Star Trek

3. Dumpling

4. Soy Sauce

5. Algorithm

6. Bambi

7. Snooker

8. Strawberry

9. Lemon

10. Hipster

11. Monster Mash

12. Meatloaf (because I would do anything for love, but I won't do that)

13. Santa Claus

14. Cornflakes (because, ironically, there is a since-debunked myth that these were created to prevent masturbation)

15. Pizza

16. Sacramento

17. Mailbox

18. Sushi

19. Marinara

20. Nicki Minaj

I think it's pretty obvious I just sat at my computer and spat these bad boys out. But this should give you a little taste of some of your options. Your safe word can literally be anything that you want.

Don't be afraid to have fun with it. If you decide to use "Meatloaf" and, upon uttering the word aloud, you decide you would rather cut off your own foot than ever use that as a safe word again, you're free to choose something else. Just remember to double and triple check with your partner(s) that you're all aware of what the safe word is before starting a scene.

You can also opt for safe gestures. Sometimes we actually can't say words—because, ahem, maybe we're wearing a ball gag or something of that nature. In this instance, a gesture would be more appropriate. Keep it simple. I like the "Three Tap Rule." If you are reaching a limit, you reach out and tap, tap, tap your partner—a little vigorously, but not *too* vigorously—and this acts as your safe word. Again, you can customize your safe gestures to fit your needs and preferences.

## SAFE WORD ACTION PLANS

You're in the middle of a very hot scene wherein you're being a Mommy Dominatrix and flogging your naughty little baby sub. Suddenly, they call the safe word. The play stops. So, now what? Follow this three-step plan.

### 1. Stop what you're doing and check in

If the safe word is called, the scene stops. In practice, it can be a bit unsettling—and even upsetting to hear a safe word. No one wants to think they've done something wrong, you know? We're in a vulnerable position during a scene, whether you're the Dom or sub. We all want our partners to feel safe and taken care of—and, you know, we want to feel like we know what we're doing.

It's important to take a breath and remember that this is not a personal attack on you. It's an opportunity to reconnect and get on the same page with your partner.

Take their hand (if you can) and lead them to a safe space. Take time to check in and figure out why the safe word was used. There are seriously endless reasons why a limit may have been reached. Stay open and stay attuned. Was this emotional overwhelm? Was something too painful? Did a certain phrase or word you used not work for them? Understanding why a safe word was called can help us create closer bonds—and make our scenes better in the long run. Endeavor to understand what your partner would need from you to feel more contained in the future. This is a learning opportunity and will make you a better kink practitioner—even if it feels uncomfortable in the moment.

## 2. Decide how you want to move forward

Once you've established why the safe word was used, collaborate on your next steps. It might just be an old "whoopsie daisy," and you can go forward and start the scene again. In fact, I would be bold enough to say that this is usually how a lot of these dynamics wind up playing out, but not always. Sometimes you hear the safe word, and the scene is now over. That's OK too. It doesn't mean you can't do that scene again in the future.

Ask your partner what they need from you to feel safe. Share your needs as well. It's incredibly important that you don't jump back into a scene for the sake of your partner. Both of you need to enter back into a kink dynamic because it's mutually agreed on and desired.

### 3. Take accountability

OK, now this one can be a toughy, I know. We have to be willing to take accountability if we cross someone's boundary. Sometimes we don't always know we have a boundary until the boundary has been crossed. We're human. We're not perfect. Nevertheless, if you cross a boundary (even if you weren't aware of it), take accountability and apologize. Do whatever your partner needs to feel safe and secure again—within reason, of course. Kink is a collaborative experience. We all play a part. Sometimes things go wrong, and that's OK as long as we hold ourselves accountable. We'll dive more into action plans for accountability later in this chapter, and you'll find an exercise at the end.

## BOUNDARIES AND LIMITS

Boundaries and limits. I keep using these words, but we need to understand what they mean. Boundaries and limits are the edges of our play. They are the lines we don't want crossed. These serve as the container for the scene. We know not to cross a boundary with our partner, and they know not to cross ours. As mentioned, we sometimes don't know a boundary is a boundary until we've reached it—hence the safe words. With that being said, we usually will have a pretty good understanding of what we do and do not want. It's OK to leave some room for that lovely "enthusiastic maybe"—but even that should be contained in the understanding that you may decide "Wow, F this very much" and call the safe word.

If you find yourself playing with someone who says they have no boundaries or don't believe in boundaries, *run* the other way.

## SETTING BOUNDARIES

Learning to set and uphold boundaries is one of the most essential skills in your kink toolbox—and honestly, it's just a crucial life skill in general. At its core, boundary setting is an act of self-awareness and self-respect. It's about truly knowing yourself: your comfort zones, your limits, your needs, and your deal-breakers. Sure, pushing your boundaries and experimenting with new sensations, roles, or dynamics can be thrilling, but exploration doesn't replace the need for emotional and physical safety. There is nothing more empowering than knowing what feels right for you, and just as importantly, knowing what doesn't.

Let's make this crystal clear: You are under no obligation to do anything you don't feel comfortable doing—ever. You are not required to kiss someone you're not attracted to. You are not obligated to try anal play just because your partner is curious. You do *not* need to perform or engage in any activity that doesn't feel like a full-bodied yes for you—full stop. And on the flip side, if someone doesn't want to engage in something that you're into, you have no right to push them, guilt them, or try to change their mind. Consent is mutual. Respect goes both ways.

This is where boundaries come in. Boundaries are an integral part of consent education and ethical kink play. Psychosexual and relationships psychotherapist Silva Neves succinctly defines a boundary as follows: "A personal boundary is the line between what is acceptable and what is unacceptable in relationships with others, with romantic and sexual partners and also with friends, family members and peers." This applies to kink partners as well.

## "EXPLICIT" VS. "IMPLICIT" BOUNDARIES

Think of boundaries as fluid, not fixed—they evolve and shift alongside your personal growth, your experiences, and your comfort levels. What felt off-limits six months ago might now feel worth exploring, and something you were once open to might no longer feel safe or exciting. This is why it's so important to keep checking in with yourself: How do I feel about this now? Has anything changed for me? Do I still want to engage with this activity or role-play?

In the world of intimacy and kink, boundaries can generally be broken down into two main categories: explicit and implicit.

Explicit boundaries are those you articulate clearly, directly, and deliberately. These are personal, self-determined rules you share with a partner, and they should be stated plainly before play even begins. For example, if choking is a no-go for you, you need to say it clearly: "Choking is not something I'm comfortable with." It might sound obvious, but because of how normalized certain acts (like choking) have become in porn and mainstream media, too many people assume something is "on the table" just because they've seen it done frequently online. Clear communication around explicit boundaries can help prevent misunderstanding, discomfort, and harm.

Implicit boundaries are the boundaries we expect others to respect based on shared social values, human rights, and commonly accepted norms—things like bodily autonomy, privacy, and the right to say no without pressure or coercion. "They are related to human rights, legal rights, and the accepted codes of socialization," Neves says.

## REAFFIRMING BOUNDARIES BEFORE, DURING, AND AFTER PLAY

Boundary setting isn't a one-time thing. It's an ongoing conversation—one that ideally happens before, during, and after any scene or intimate interaction. Before you engage in any play, take the time to have a meaningful talk about your boundaries. These discussions can happen in person, over text, or even as part of a pre-scene checklist. Whatever method works for you is valid, as long as it's happening.

Aftercare is just as important a time to revisit those boundaries. Check in with yourself and with your partner(s): Did anything come up that you weren't expecting? Did a boundary get tested or crossed, intentionally or unintentionally? Do you need to shift your limits now that you've had that experience?

"During the conversation, you can explore all the pleasurable things you love, and clearly state that the things you don't love are off the table," says Lorrae Bradbury, a sex coach and founder of the sex-positive site, Slutty Girl Problems. "You don't need to explain your reasons or context for your boundaries. Your boundaries are valid and don't require any further explanation. There's no need to apologize for setting a boundary." Let's repeat that for the people in the back: You don't need to apologize for your boundaries. You don't owe anyone a reason. Your "No" doesn't need a backstory. It is reason enough on its own.

If you communicate a boundary and your partner ignores it or violates it, that is a serious red flag. If someone disregards your clearly communicated limits—whether by accident or intentionally—they're showing you that they may not be a safe or respectful person to play with. If you've said, "I don't like being called a slut during play," and your partner continues to do it, that's a breach of your boundary and it needs to be addressed, directly and firmly. If someone repeatedly disregards your boundaries, it's no longer just a misunderstanding—it's disrespect at best, and potentially coercion or assault at worst.

In the event of a boundary violation, stop the scene immediately. "Don't be afraid to stop it. It is essential," Neves explains. "Then you explain explicitly that it was a breach of boundaries and ask them with more assertiveness to remember it and not do it again."

Be assertive and clear in naming what happened. You might say something like "I've told you before that being called a slut crosses a line for me. You've now violated that boundary. This cannot happen again—do you understand?"

If they continue to push your limits or dismiss your discomfort, take that as a cue to walk away. You deserve partners who take your boundaries seriously.

## HARD LIMITS VS. SOFT LIMITS

Gigi is at it again with the nuance, folx! Let's talk about hard limits and soft limits. Not everything is as simple as it seems in Kink Land. Sure, we all have boundaries and limits, but not every limit is set in stone. We can think of limits as falling on a spectrum, much like the kink spectrum. On one end, we have no limits, and on the other, we have hard limits—with soft limits falling somewhere in the general direction of hard limits, but not quite.

### Hard limits

A hard limit is an absolute boundary. It is immovable, unchangeable, and set in stone. A hard limit is something that is out of bounds for someone. For example, a hard limit might be caning. You're completely unwilling to even toy with the idea of being caned by your partner. You are not into it, and it's not going to be on the table in a scene, under any circumstances.

Hard limits can take on a myriad of different forms. They can be phrases, certain acts, certain objects, or certain scene dynamics. You may decide you're here for leather, but using latex in a scene is a hard limit. You might like being called a "filthy pig boy," but being told you're a good boy is a hard limit.

Of course, now that I've made these bold claims about hard limits being set in stone, let me fuck with your head: Sometimes hard limits can shift into soft limits—or stop being limits at all. We're all different, and for some of us, our boundaries change. It's important that we continually look at our hard limits and reflect on them in order to gain better self-understanding. Maybe your hard limits will change; maybe they won't. Maybe they'll shift into something different, or maybe they won't. Either way, it's all good as long as you're playing in a way that feels safe and authentic to you.

What is important to remember is that in the present moment, if a partner states something is a hard limit, it isn't a negotiation. That is the hard limit, and it is to be respected and honored.

### Soft limits

Soft limits are like the fuzzy gray areas around our comfort zones: We know the edge is near, but we're not sure just how near. A soft limit is when you're at a boundary, but you might be willing to play or experiment with that boundary. This can apply to acts or objects being used only in certain contexts, with certain partners, or in specific ways.

For example, you might find pain play to be a limit for you, but you're willing to experiment with it. Maybe you like a bit of light spanking, but anything other than that is a hard limit. Another example might be butt play. Maybe you're not into it all the time, but are willing to lightly play with it under the right circumstances or with very specific toys.

Basically, soft limits boil down to limits that have wiggle room. They aren't set in stone, but they are still boundaries. Sometimes playing with your softer limits can be exciting, while also generating a bit of fear. As long as everyone is being safe and intentional, we can play with our edges safely. Check out the "exploring soft limits" exercise for more.

Understanding our boundaries and limits is so crucial in playing with kink safely. We should endeavor to honor our partner—and to honor ourselves. Remember, your boundaries are valid and they deserve to be respected. Hopefully, you feel more solid about how boundaries work and how to set them. You're doing such a great job!

## PLAYING WITH BOUNDARIES

Boundaries are the edges, and sometimes playing with the edges is fun. We often want to push ourselves to the limit, and this is sexy as hell. In kink, you may decide to play up to the very edge of a boundary or tolerance. This is completely OK to do—assuming you've negotiated this with a partner and have the safe word ready to go at any time. In these instances, the safe word is used to indicate when you've reached the boundary and can't take any more.

For example, tickle play. This play is appealing to people who get sexually aroused by tickling. This might be in fetish or kink form, and will vary from person to person. In tickle play (or tickle torture, as it's sometimes called), you may decide with your partner that you want them to tie you up and tickle you to the point where you can't take it anymore. You have a boundary (when you can't take it anymore), but you're not sure exactly where the boundary will come up. Tickling is a great way to play with boundaries because there is very little chance anyone could get harmed by this action—you know, just as a suggestion!

Playing with the edges of your comfort zone is one of the things that makes kink play so much fun. Just remember to communicate, have your safe word ready, and continuously check in with your partner.

## ACTION PLANS FOR ACCOUNTABILITY

Mistakes happen during scenes. We know this. We're human beings. If we cross a boundary, make someone angry, triggered, or upset, or even just land that spank wrong or tie the ties too tight, we need to be accountable. Having a boundary crossed can be especially frightening and triggering for some folx. Good kink partners are willing to be accountable for their missteps and take appropriate reparative measures where needed. While everyone can become emotionally overwhelmed, triggered, or scared during a scene, this might be even more likely for neurodivergent partners who may experience overstimulation in certain contexts.

The thing is, we mess up sometimes. The way toward better experiences is in how we deal with it. Follow these simple steps to compassionately hold yourself and your partners accountable for boundary violations, accidental triggers, and mistakes.

Now, before we jump into the steps, I want to make one thing very clear: When we're talking about a boundary violation, we are talking about a mistake. This means it was not intentional to harm the other person. We are *not* talking about abuse. If you did intentionally cross someone's boundary, yes, you do need to be accountable, but chances are there is no going back from such a deep level of betrayal, because intentionally crossing someone's explicit boundaries and limits is sexual assault.

### Step 1: Stop what you're doing and check in

If you:

* hear the safe word

* see that your partner isn't responding in the way they normally would

* think the vibe is off...

*Stop* what you are doing and check in. A person can be in such an intense nervous system response that they cannot communicate normally. We call this a "freeze" response. It's a survival response wherein your nervous system truly believes that shutting down is the best chance you have at not dying. It's some lizard-brain-level stuff. If you think something is off, check in with your partner. As we've said in previous chapters, one of the most important parts of being in a D/s dynamic is attunement to your partner.

### Step 2: Listen compassionately

Find out what went wrong. Be open and compassionate. If there was a boundary violation, try to stay attuned and take in what is being said with open ears.

Remember, don't get defensive—reflect instead. This isn't a

reflection of you as a person. You made a mistake, and that's OK. But going on the defensive instead of taking in what your partner is saying and integrating that feedback is not going to benefit you. It could lead to further ruptures in your relationship.

### Step 3: Apologize (and mean it)

If you accidentally harm someone, you need to apologize. And you need to mean it. When screw-ups happen and someone ends up being collateral, you have to be willing to own the mistake.

You're also welcome to offer how this experience has made you feel with intention. Now is not the time for "you" statements. It's time to use "I" statements. It's not conducive to good communication to say, "Well, *you* did this thing and that's why I did that thing." Instead, try: "When this happened/when you did this thing, it made me feel X way." Part of accountability is understanding the role we play and taking ownership of our emotions, rather than making it all about blame and finger-pointing.

### Step 4: Make repairs where needed

Find out from your partner what they need to feel safe with you. Keep in mind that not every partner will be willing to do repair work. They may decide not to play with you again—and that is their right. If you can make repairs, try to do what is needed—within reason, of course. This can look like having deep conversations, reworking your boundaries, trying a different kind of play than the one where the mistake happened, going to therapy together, and much more. The important thing here is not to ignore the mistake and try to bury it. Facing our mistakes head-on and with conviction can bring about stronger healing.

## Step 5: Learn from your mistakes

If you crossed a boundary, don't do it again. Learn from your mistakes and move forward with greater knowledge. This may look like better listening, taking more kink courses, or simply learning better attunement. Messing something up doesn't mean you're banned from kink for life. You can take the wisdom of past missteps and move forward with greater knowledge and empathy.

---

### Chapter 12 recap

In Chapter 12, we created the kink container and provided some ways for you to start constructing your own. We looked at the wonderful world of safe words and why they're so important. I gave you 20 fun and interesting safe words to try out—because why not?

Next, we outlined boundaries and limits, making distinctions between explicit and implicit boundaries, as well as hard and soft limits.

Last, we explored the tricky and often very tender role of accountability when it comes to boundary violations, with actionable steps you can take to heal a wrong, however unintentional.

---

## JOURNAL PROMPTS

1. Consider a boundary you've had in the past that has changed over time. This doesn't have to be a sexual or kinky boundary, but it certainly can be. Reflect on how this boundary has

shifted and changed over time. Why do you think that is? What does this change mean for you and your current way of living?

2.  Think about a time someone crossed a boundary with you. What was that experience like? What did you do—or not do—about it? How do you feel about it now? Please take care when doing this reflection, as it has the potential to bring up difficult feelings or memories. If you feel this one is too much for you, feel free to skip it.

3.  Think about a soft limit and a hard limit. What makes the soft limit soft? What does that even mean for you? What makes your hard limit feel so immovable?

4.  Consider a form of play—or a sex act—that was once a hard limit and shifted into something you've enjoyed. If you can't think of anything, take some time to reflect on why that might be. Get curious!

## EXERCISES

### EXERCISE 1: Safe words in the wild game

The purpose of this exercise is to help you listen for and catch a safe word. Safe words need to trigger us into action—to help us know a limit has been reached and play needs to stop. Practice can help build attunement.

First things first: Choose your safe word. Take some time to think it through and decide on something that works for you. Then, ask your partner or a friend to practice with you out in the real world, not during sex. When you're out and about, try using the safe word. This should stop all activity that is currently taking place. Get creative with it.

For example, your safe word is "caramel." You're walking with your friend down the street, talking about what you did yesterday. Suddenly, you drop in the word "caramel." All conversation should stop, and you should both freeze.

If your friend catches the safe word, they get a point. If they don't, you get a point. The first to receive five points wins. Then, switch turns.

## EXERCISE 2: Defining your limits and boundaries

Pop out your Yes, No, Maybe list from Chapter 9. Next to each option, write H (hard limit), N (no limit), or S (soft limit). Below, write down a few limits that might not be on the list. Take some time to reflect on these different limits and consider where they fall on the Hard to Soft Spectrum—and why. Remember that context may be important. For instance, a cock cage may be a hard limit, but with a specific partner, it can be something you enjoy. Take your time with this one and come back to it, as needed.

## EXERCISE 3: Exploring soft limits

Choose a soft limit that you feel particularly comfortable with. Either with a partner or on your own, explore that limit. Start by reflecting on it. Journaling about it can help.

Then, explore bringing that soft limit into a fantasy. You can talk it through with a partner, imagine it in your head during self-pleasure, or even try it out in real life with a partner. Take it slowly and be sure to check in with yourself. Don't be afraid to invoke the safe word, even if you're using it with yourself.

When you've finished the exercise, take some time to reflect once again. Has anything changed? Did you learn anything about this limit or yourself in doing this exercise?

Now, on to one of my favorite things of all when it comes to kink: aftercare.

# 13

## YOUR GUIDE TO AFTERCARE

### What you'll find in this chapter:

→ Why aftercare?

→ Aftercare and kink.

→ Aftercare and the impact on partner bonding.

→ What does aftercare entail?

→ Creating your aftercare plan to come down from scenes in an emotionally safe way.

→ The Golden Rules of Aftercare.

→ Agony Aunt question and answer.

→ Exercises.

**A**ftercare refers to the time we devote, post-sex or play, to cuddle, talk, and care for each other. You may think this is simply "what you do after sex," but it has important implications. In the kink community, aftercare is essential. When a couple comes down from the highs of BDSM play, there can be an emotional crash. The dominant partner must provide aftercare for the submissive partner for them to feel at ease and ready to rejoin the real world.

While we're talking about kink here (obviously), it's not just the kinky folx who can benefit from a connecting and grounding post-play experience together. In my own practice, I'm a big proponent of *all* couples devoting time to post-euphoric aftercare to rekindle closeness, regardless of the play they engage in. Whether you're strapping your partner to a St. Andrew's cross for a whipping or having sex in the missionary position, aftercare should still be a part of the routine.

## WHY AFTERCARE?

But, Gigi, you might be thinking, I just wanted to get my ass beaten and then go home. I barely know this person. Why should I have to stay and, like, get emotionally settled? Why should I invest in this other person's well-being when I may never even see them again?

Well, because you might consider this to be a casual, non-committed, super fun little adventure—but your nervous system doesn't, and the same goes for your partner.

Whether we want to admit it or not, sexually charged experiences come with heightened emotional states. It doesn't matter if the experience is casual or part of a committed relationship, kinky, vanilla, or while wearing penguin onesies; when we get down and dirty, there are going to be emotions involved. How could there not be?

When we get into intense erotic states, our brains are flooded with a ton of neurochemicals like adrenaline, dopamine, and oxytocin. Desire is a complex biological and psychological state. As such, when we reach climax (or the end of the sexual experience), we need to be sure we get back to a healthy and relaxed mental state. Simply throwing your clothes on and going about your day, without so much as a "thanks for the good times, pal," doesn't work for most people.

This is why aftercare is such a crucial component of sexual play. Aftercare is the post-sex scaffolding that allows us to walk away from a sexual experience or kink scene feeling good about ourselves. Zachary Zane, author of *Boyslut* and by now our well-known pal, tells me that aftercare has "typically been associated with kink or particularly 'intense' sexual scenes, though engaging in aftercare shouldn't be limited to solely kinky or BDSM experiences."

Aftercare has its place in all forms of sex. This is just something to keep in mind as we're moving through your kink journey. It's a good idea to start practicing aftercare now, before kink is even on the table. I can assure you that it will make your sexual experiences better.

## AFTERCARE AND KINK

"Aftercare exists because doing a scene can be very intense, taking you into a super activated state of consciousness," certified sex coach and clinical sexologist Lucy Rowett tells me in an interview: "Intensity of any kind, be it pleasurable, painful, or the delicious line between both, is incredibly overstimulating."

Because of this overstimulation, it is important to consider the ways you're going to bring yourself and your partner back down into a state of calm once play concludes. A lot of us don't consider the aftermath when we're engaging in sex, but failing to do so can lead to less-than or even shitty experiences. "Often, what happens *after* the sexual experience impacts how we view the experience," Zane explains. "For example, if you had *incredible* sex, but [they kick] you to the curb the moment they orgasm, you're likely not going to view the experience fondly. You'll just remember feeling used, rushed, and kicked out." No one deserves to feel this way, ever.

This inattention (neglect, even) can lead to "sub drop" or "Top drop," which we've talked about already in the context of the post-coital blues. You can be left feeling depressed, anxious, and even used. When we take time to check in, acknowledge our humanity and feelings, and feel seen and heard, we're setting ourselves up to cope better with the emotional plummet. It's just basic common decency, folx. I know this is a foreign concept in the age of hookup culture, but we need to leave this "love 'em and leave 'em" mentality in the bin. It isn't good for anyone. If you're having sex, doing kink, and sharing erotic experiences, emotions are present, and connection happens. Sorry, I can't be cool and pretend this isn't the case—but it isn't.

## AFTERCARE AND PARTNER BONDING

If you're in a relationship—or multiple relationships—aftercare isn't just a nice extra; it's one of the most powerful tools you have for deepening intimacy, nurturing trust, and building a stronger emotional foundation with your partner(s). Great sex and wild kink scenes might feel exhilarating in the moment, but a lasting connection is forged in what comes after—in the tender, quiet moments of closeness, care, and emotional regulation that help both partners land gently back on solid ground.

Aftercare isn't just about cleaning up the toys or getting a glass of water (though both of those things are excellent!). It's about intentionally tending to the emotional, physical, and psychological state of your partner—and yourself—after a scene or sexual experience. It's about being present, showing compassion, and acknowledging that intimate play, no matter how casual or intense, impacts our nervous systems and emotional well-being. And when done right, aftercare can create an incredible opportunity for bonding and connection that actually enhances future play and deepens your relationship dynamic overall.

Couples who engage in thoughtful, consistent aftercare often develop a stronger sense of closeness and attunement than those who don't. Why? Because after sex or kink play, we're at our most raw. We're physically exposed, emotionally open, and awash in a potent cocktail of neurochemicals like oxytocin, dopamine, and serotonin. Our bodies are buzzing, but our emotional systems may still be catching up. That's exactly why aftercare is essential—it helps anchor us in connection and safety when we're in a post-play, post-orgasm haze.

"Everyone feels good when they know their partner cares for them, and what better way to show it than by tending to them when they are in a vulnerable post-sex state of mind?" explains licensed psychotherapist and couples therapist Pam Saffer, LMFT.

"Prioritizing time [for] aftercare provides space to improve emotional intimacy, sharing, and validating positive emotions. It really encourages couples to share open communication and express love [and] kindness towards each other either verbally or through affectionate touch," Kristine D'Angelo, a certified sex coach and clinical sexologist, explained in an interview.

Aftercare isn't reserved for long-term relationships or committed partnerships. It doesn't matter whether you're married, dating, casually hooking up, in a one-night stand, or engaging in a play scene with a new kink partner—it still matters. Everyone deserves to feel safe, grounded, and respected after a vulnerable encounter.

Take time to connect with your partner(s) and reflect gently and positively on what just unfolded between you. Say kind words. Validate their experience. Offer reassurance if anything felt intense or vulnerable. Let them know you appreciate them. Let them know they're safe with you. You'll be amazed at how much more vibrant your connection can become.

## WHAT AFTERCARE ENTAILS

Aftercare is as unique as the sexual experience itself. It can include talking, cuddling, comparing notes on the experience, having a snack, watching a show, playing with your partner's hair, going off to have a breather alone, taking a shower alone/together, etc., etc., etc. There is no limit to the menu of activities you have to choose from.

Aftercare also "involves practical things like tending to any bruises or cuts that you sustained during the scene, cleaning up the place, and even kissing it better," Rowett says. "It needs to be something you find comforting and soothing, ideally that involves something restful."

The way aftercare plays out is completely subjective and will depend on the needs and desires of everyone involved in the play.

Zane tells us that aftercare is really about caring for the emotional well-being of the people you play with. "At its core, you're asking your partner how they're feeling and if there's anything they need from you," he says. "They may want to cuddle, a glass of water, to share something that triggered them during sex, or something else entirely."

## CREATING AN AFTERCARE PLAN TO COME DOWN IN AN EMOTIONALLY SAFE WAY

Knowing what you need as aftercare is a part of understanding yourself as a sexual being. This means considering what your needs are post-sex, not just during sex.

Ask yourself these questions:

1. What did my last great sexual experience look like?

2. What do I want right after sex that I've been afraid to ask for?

3. What would make me feel safe and cared for after sex?

You'll find these questions stated again in the journal prompts section, so you have space to reflect.

It doesn't matter if you met your partner on an app 30 minutes ago; you still deserve to get the aftercare you need. If a person refuses to meet your aftercare needs, you may want to reconsider whether this is someone you feel safe enough to play with.

It's important to consider where your aftercare needs intersect and where they differ. This requires open and honest communication with your partner. "If one of you needs a long cuddle afterwards but the other needs alone time, you will need to make this clear and negotiate a way in the middle," Rowett says.

While directly asking how your partner is feeling is very important, Zane points out that aftercare can also mean taking a few minutes to decompress before verbally checking in after sex. "Simply being with that person and holding them is a form of aftercare. After a few minutes, you can ask how they're feeling," he says.

Last, aftercare isn't always about the "right here, right now." It can often extend into the next day. "You can send a text asking how they're feeling or if there's anything they need from you," Zane adds.

What all this juicy stuff boils down to is caring for the welfare of someone who shared an experience with you. We're all just humans trying to find joy, pleasure, and comfort with the people we engage with. Every person we have sex with has a right to a good experience, and this includes emotional safety, too.

## THE TEN GOLDEN RULES OF AFTERCARE

### 1. Discuss aftercare before play

As with all negotiations involving sex and kink, conversations about aftercare should be clearly outlined before you start playing. This way, you can be confident that your needs will be met and respected—this goes for your partner, too. These conversations can happen in person, over the phone, or via text—whatever is easiest for you. It can also be helpful to do a quick check-in and go over the plan in person right before you jump into a scene.

### 2. Get crystal clear on what you need

Getting the aftercare you want and need requires knowing exactly *what* you want and asking for it. It can be helpful to start with Exercise 1 in the exercises section to think through what you want from aftercare. This way, you have a list ready to go.

### 3. Don't judge your partner's aftercare needs

We all deserve empathy, consideration, and respect. If your partner needs something you consider "unusual" or "weird," etc., you shouldn't be a dick about it. We all need different things to feel safe and contained after play. Remember, you're both in a vulnerable state, and it takes a lot of courage to voice your needs. If their request is something you're truly not comfortable doing, you can say, "I'm not really comfortable with that activity, exactly. Is there an alternative that might work for you?" Collaborate and find a solution.

### 4. Openly discuss what you're feeling after the scene

Having some time to talk through the scene can be very helpful for grounding and coming back to reality. Being open and honest can contribute to feeling safe. This includes acknowledging any difficult emotions you may be experiencing and asking for reassurance where needed.

### 5. Set up an aftercare station or space

Consider the ambiance of an aftercare station. It will look different for everyone based on personal preferences, but generally speaking, you want to consider:

- low lighting (I personally *love* fairy lights for an aftercare space—they're just so calming)

- comfortable furniture and blankets

- pleasing scents (such as candles or reed diffusers)

- relaxing music or white noise

- any equipment you might need—such as a first-aid kit, a hot water kettle, and tea bags, etc.

And once play concludes, aftercare should take place immediately. You need to move from being in the scene to being in the recovery space.

### 6. Be willing to walk away if you're not aligned with your partner

This is an annoying one, I know. If your partner is unwilling to collaborate with you on your aftercare plan—or doesn't respect your aftercare plan once play concludes—you need to be willing to walk away. If they don't prioritize making you feel safe and centered after play, they just aren't a safe person to play with. It's as simple as that, babe.

Do not compromise your mental well-being to please someone else, no matter how great the orgasms are.

### 7. Check in with your play partner the next day (and even in the days that follow)

No matter how casual a play partner is—even if you're only ever going to play that one time—always check in with a text or phone call the next day to make sure they're feeling good and to let them know you had a nice time (assuming you did have a nice time). You can say:

- I had a fun time playing yesterday. Just wanted to be sure you're feeling alright. How are you?

- Hi! Just wanted to check in and make sure you're feeling good after the scene yesterday. I know play can be intense sometimes.

- Are you feeling OK after yesterday? I get pretty bad sub drop/ Top drop sometimes, so I just wanted to be sure you're feeling alright.

We all deserve to be treated like whole human beings, and we all deserve to have our feelings cared for.

### 8. Discuss boundaries (new and old) for the next time you meet

If you're planning to meet up again or make this a more regular thing, go over your boundaries each time before you play. Our boundaries are not fixed. They are always shifting. So, when we play with someone new, try something different, or even if we're with someone we know very well and are doing familiar play, we may find something doesn't work for us anymore (or that we're curious to try something different). Having ongoing conversations as a part of aftercare can help you make sure you're both/all getting what you want out of each play session.

### 9. Have a self-care aftercare plan in place for after play

Aftercare doesn't end just because you're on your own again. Consider some relaxing, grounding solo activities you can do when you get home (or when you're finished with your play) to take care of yourself. This can include taking a bath, reading a book, cooking a nice meal, watching a favorite movie, and so forth. Intentionally caring for our well-being—rather than mindlessly scrolling through our phones—can help us avoid feeling those pesky sad feelings that can come post-play.

## 10. Change your aftercare plan as needed

Just like with boundaries, aftercare needs also shift and change with time and context. If something you once enjoyed (or thought you'd enjoy) doesn't work for you, be willing to shift and change your activities accordingly.

**AGONY AUNT QUESTION AND ANSWER: I have a lot of problems with "sub drop." What can I do to help?**

**Q** *Dear Gigi,*

*I've been in the kink world for a long while, but have only recently started playing casually with people. Before, I was in a relationship for about three years, where we did a lot of fun kink scenes. The relationship didn't work out for a lot of reasons—mostly to do with the fact that I viewed them much more as a friend, but didn't know how to pull myself out once I was committed.*

*Anyways, while I've been having a great time, I find that after a casual encounter, I feel really, really bad. I feel used, gross, and generally like the only thing I have to offer is my body and sex. Usually, we have sex and/or a scene of some kind, and then we get dressed and go about our lives.*

*Which is what I want, I think?*

*I'm not sure if this is because I'm overly sensitive or if casual sex just isn't for me. What should I do? This is messing with my ability to have good kink experiences, and I'd like to get myself out of it.*

*Sensitive Submissive*

A Dear Sensitive Submissive,

I believe what you're expressing is "sub drop." It's very, very common. I'd love to start by breaking it down because I think understanding what is going on for you could help figure out ways to get through it.

When a sub gets into a scene, they can slip into a state of mind called subspace. This is akin to a meditative experience. Emotions and endorphins run high. But what comes up must come down, honey. Since being in subspace is a highly emotive experience, it can come along with a post-session crash in the minutes, hours, or days following an intense scene. When all the happy and feel-good chemicals wear off, we can experience an emotional drop.

When we experience sub drop, we might feel anxious, depressed, disoriented, and other not-great feelings. I suspect this is what you're going through.

Sub drop can look similar to post-coital dysphoria (PCD)—also known as the post-sex blues. It's believed to come from the euphoric rush and sudden come-down that follows intense sexual pleasure. It is the brain's way of recalibrating. Research has shown that nearly half of people have experienced PCD at some point in their lives.

Aftercare is the salve that soothes these sad feelings. Sometimes we can feel isolated or disconnected from our partners after sex, once all those lovely, juicy feelings of pleasure wear off. This is why "aftercare" is so important in BDSM. We need an aftercare routine to ensure both parties are able to return to a sense of psychological equilibrium.

How you practice aftercare will depend on your needs. It can look like cuddling, making a cup of tea, taking a hot shower, talking about what happened during the scene, and more. It's about creating a safe and comforting place to calm down and feel settled after such emotional highs.

I get that the experiences you're having are casual—and that's great for you!—but that doesn't mean you don't need or deserve aftercare, babe.

Have an open and honest discussion about how you tend to feel after scenes and develop an aftercare routine that makes you feel safe and secure. You might want to cuddle, or perhaps you want your partner to stroke your arm, or you might want to have a nice chat or a deeper conversation. This should all be discussed in pre-play negotiations. If a partner isn't willing to give you these things, they aren't someone to play with. A seasoned kinkster will know how important aftercare is and will be more than happy to accommodate.

If you know there is a specific thing or activity that helps you settle after a particularly intense scene (or any scene, really), don't be afraid to speak up and ask for it. Our partners—no matter how casual or serious—should want us to feel safe and secure after scenes. If you're playing with someone who doesn't show interest in you feeling safe and secure, they are unlikely to be a very safe person. If this is the case, I would not recommend playing with them again.

Sex is very fun, but it can be an emotionally fraught thing in addition to all the pleasures, so we need to take precautions to ensure that everyone walks away from the experience feeling positive and good about themselves. Whatever form of aftercare works for you is perfectly fine. Just be sure you discuss it before any sexy time takes place. When it comes to sex, we all deserve to walk out the door afterwards feeling emotionally whole and great about ourselves.

I hope this helps. Casual sex and kink may or may not be for you—only you get to make that call! But I truly think that with a little aftercare and TLC, you'll probably find that this is a lot more fun than you expected. You've got this.

XOXO Auntie Gigi

Well, there we have it—everything you need to know about aftercare. You've come so far! I'm so proud of you.

### Chapter 13 recap

In Chapter 13, we explored the importance of aftercare and why we need it in all forms of play, intimacy, and sex. We considered aftercare's place in kink play, specifically, and why it is such an integral part of getting kinky. We also looked at how aftercare can impact long-term relationships and partner bonding. Aftercare is the stuff that keeps us grounded and feeling good when we're engaging in the intense emotional highs of kink play and sex. It always has its place and should be honored.

Next, we took some time to break down what aftercare entails and what it can look like in practice. Everyone will be different and will need different things, but aftercare is all about engaging in activities that help you feel safe, comfortable, and grounded after play.

Then, we considered what it might look like to create your own aftercare plan, to come down from scenes in an emotionally safe way—lots of things to think about there! Figuring out what works for you takes self-reflection and compassion.

Next, we explored the Ten Golden Rules of Aftercare. These should act as a guide for all kink players to ensure everyone feels great after they play.

Last, we broke down a question from a reader who was wondering how to deal with sub drop—and if their low emotional states after casual play meant they weren't cut out for casual experiences.

## JOURNAL PROMPTS

1. What did my last great sexual experience look like?

2. What do I want right after sex that I've been afraid to ask for?

3. What would make me feel safe and cared for after sex? You can choose to simply list the activities that you believe would work for you.

4. If I find that I'm still feeling low after play, how can my partner best support me? What changes can I make (or things can I add) to my aftercare activities that may help?

5. What are three self-care things I can do for myself to get

grounded after a scene, when I'm on my own? (Take a bath, read my favorite book, watch my comfort show, cook a lovely meal, go for a walk, etc.)

# EXERCISES

### EXERCISE 1: Aftercare activities that work for you

**Step 1:** Get out your colored pencils, crayons, or colored pens. Write down activities you:

*   enjoy (green)

*   find comforting (pink)

*   find relaxing (blue)

*   find make you feel safe (yellow)

*   find calm you down when you're in a heightened state (purple).

Try doing these in different colors in order to figure out which feelings each activity brings about for you. Ask yourself: What emotions and feelings do I experience that make me enjoy this activity? You can also write down activities and circle them with corresponding colors if they bring out multiple emotional states.

**Step 2:** Decide which of these activities you think would work with a partner involved and underline them. This will help you narrow down exactly what activities you want to be a part of your aftercare plan.

**Step 3:** Distill these down further by then breaking your activities into "long-term partner," "casual partner," and "ongoing play partner" to denote which activities would work for you, given the level of intimacy and closeness you have with specific partners.

**EXERCISE 2:** Mapping out your aftercare plan

**Step 1:** Write down one to five things you *enjoy* having as a part of aftercare.

**Step 2:** Write down one to five things you *require* as part of aftercare. Some of these may overlap with the items from Step 1. If they do, circle or highlight the things that are most important to you.

**Step 3:** Write down one to five things you do *not* want during after-care—whether they be things your partner does or you do.

**Step 4:** Write down one to five things you can do after you leave your partner to take care of yourself.

**Step 5:** Choose three main things that you'd like to have as a part of your aftercare plan. This can be shared with any potential partners you plan to play with. Ask your partner to share their aftercare must-haves with you, too. There just might be some overlap!

*Sidenote:* It can be helpful to draw these maps out as well. Whatever works for you—do that!

**Step 6:** Collaborate with your partner on *how* you're going to execute aftercare so both of you feel taken care of. This can include figuring out the order of activities, asking how each person would like the activity to look, and checking in throughout the aftercare experience.

# 14

# BRINGING A PARTNER INTO YOUR KINK JOURNEY

## What you'll find in this chapter:

→ How to talk about kink: conversational consent and holding space with empathy.

→ What to do if you need to explore your kink, but your partner isn't into it.

→ Figuring out shared kinks and where to compromise.

→ How to prepare for a "no" or "maybe."

→ How to get started with kink scenes that involve a partner:

- having conversations about where you land on the Dom/sub scale

- talking about fantasy

- starting your play slowly and intentionally.

→ Agony Aunt question and answer.

→ Conversation starters.

→ Exercises.

**Y**ou've come so far on your journey of exploration—so the question becomes: What's next? Well, bringing your partner in on the fun, of course!

This chapter will be short and sweet compared to some of the others, but it's going to be fun. This one is about wrapping up what you've learned and taking it into your life. You have so many exercises and resources at your disposal now that can be used with your partner—think: Yes, No, Maybe lists, the BDSM/kink personality test, the fantasy vs. in real life pros and cons list, etc. Not to mention your many, many journal prompts that you shouldn't hesitate to use as conversation starters. But there is more to come, too, because we have to know where to start when it comes to playing with someone else, especially if your partner is not kinky (or hasn't indicated as such).

Whether your partner is an openly kinky person, an apprehensive beginner, or someone who might not be kinky at all, I've got all the best tips, tools, and advice to take you to the mountain—and that mountain is made of leather, probably.

## HOW TO TALK ABOUT KINK: CONVERSATIONAL CONSENT AND HOLDING SPACE WITH EMPATHY

To talk about kink openly and honestly with a partner, we have to bring together everything we've learned about consent. And this includes having consent to have a conversation about potentially triggering or anxiety-provoking things. Now, I'd wager the majority of people are going to be very into the idea of trying some fun, kinky adventures—but we can't bank on that, you know?

So, the first thing you need to do is ask your partner if they're open to having a conversation about kink. You're highly resourced now, so it should be easier to talk about these topics with some authority. You can even show them this book, if you're open to reading it together.

Three ways to open a conversation around kink:

1. Are you in a place to discuss our sex life? I'd really love it if we could talk openly about fantasy together. Are you game for that?

2. I hope you'll be open to hearing this, but I'd love to maybe talk about trying some new and fun things in the bedroom. I love our sex life, and I'd love to expand it!

3. Our sex life is so important to me, and I know you feel the same way. Are you down to talk about some ways we can explore more together?

Just like the advice I gave my reader, Unsure Sub, in Chapter 9: Have these conversations outside of the bedroom. Sexual situations are too highly charged for talking about sex or kink. These are very vulnerable conversations that require a calm, non-sexual environment.

When I asked BDSM expert Dr. Celina Criss what she suggested for partners navigating the heady conversations surrounding kink, she told me that the conversation should start slowly. "You can invite questions and follow their lead, but it's also OK to be direct when talking about your desires," she says. "Acknowledge their possible discomfort and yours, if you're feeling nervous, but let them know you want to talk with them about something important to you." Always ask for empathy and understanding from your partner.

When I posed the same question to licensed sex therapist Moushumi Ghose, she told me something I found surprising—that it may be wise to avoid using terms such as "kinky" if you think that your partner may be turned off or uncomfortable with a word that can carry so much social stigma. "Instead, you can just ask them if they would ever be interested in sharing and exploring together some things that you find arousing," she explains. This can be a good place to get the conversation going in a way that doesn't freak them the F out.

Even though this conversation might be scary, it can be really necessary and even fruitful if this is something you really want to be a part of your life, which by now you should know.

What's more, even if your partner doesn't share the same interests, it doesn't automatically mean they won't be open to participating in them. "The kink might not be a turn-on for the vanilla person in the same way that it is for the kinky one, but as long as there's consent, the vanilla person can certainly derive satisfaction from their partner's enjoyment," sex and relationships therapist Rea Pearson told me.

Criss also recommends sharing *When Someone You Love Is Kinky* by Dossie Easton with your partner, as it is an in-depth guide to having a kinky partner when you are not kinky. I definitely suggest it, too. It's one of my favorite pieces of work on kink. You can never have too many resources!

## FIGURING OUT SHARED KINKS AND WAYS TO COMPROMISE

The more common ground we can find with our partners, the better the outcome will be. Invite your partner to the table. Ask them what they are into sexually. The "Creating a kinky sex menu" exercise at the end of this chapter can be really helpful for this.

"We all have our own kinks and understanding what it means to have a kink may make this more palatable for those who consider themselves to be more 'vanilla,'" Ghose says. "Sometimes it's just a matter of finding the language, and having permission to be able to express yourself sexually in a way that feels taboo."

Meeting in the middle can be crucial here. For instance, Pearson says, "If the kinky partner wants to do something particularly messy, and the vanilla person is reluctant to make a mess because of the effort required in cleaning up afterwards, the kinky person can offer to do all the cleaning." Think cake sitting, anal play, and sploshing fetishes.

## BEING PREPARED FOR A "NO" OR "MAYBE" OR A…"FUCK NO"

OK, so here is something that really can happen: Your partner may not be down to engage in your kinks at all. This is their right. We cannot force people to do things that they aren't willing to do. Consent is a must.

You've had the conversation, and they say, "No way!" What now?

If they aren't into kink, it's time to negotiate ways you can have your needs met in other ways, especially if your kinks are fundamental to your ongoing happiness and sexual wellness. "You can explore opening up to include a kinky partner," Criss explains. "Boundaries will be key. Make sure you and your partner establish agreements about what is/is not OK, how you will communicate about the extra-relationship activities, and even develop a plan for what to do if something goes not-according-to-plan."

Ghose says that an unwillingness to even entertain the idea of exploring sexually can be a sign of bigger problems within the relationship. "A lot of times in relationships there will be an unwillingness to budge, an unwillingness to accommodate one's partner's needs because they make you feel uncomfortable, while simultaneously holding them to a very firm monogamous frame," she says. If this is the case, it's important to ask for help.

Luckily, there are professionals who can help you, because reading a few books might not be enough to get you both where you need to be to accommodate this.

There are a few different kinds of sexuality professionals who can assist in helping you and your partner in establishing a stronger connection where all of your needs are met.

### 1. If your partner is willing to explore kink with you: A sex coach who specializes in kink

A sex coach is a professional who can help you explore different ways to have your needs met within the boundaries of your relationship. They "could support you and your partner in negotiating your relationship agreements and/or exploring kink together, if that is what you both desire," Criss says.

### 2. If your partner isn't willing to do kink, but wants you to be able to explore yourself: A professional BDSM practitioner

Pearson says that hiring a professional BDSM practitioner may be a good way to get your needs met. Having consent from your partner is a must, though. Professionals can also act as educators. "Many Doms are happy to educate vanilla partners in imaginative ways that they can satisfy their kinky other half, without the vanilla person having to do anything that they aren't comfortable with," Pearson adds.

### 3. If your partner outright refuses to even engage with this stuff at all: A sex therapist who is kink-affirming

If your partner is not willing to allow you to engage with your kinks in any way, you should consider going to a sex therapist, because this is indicative of larger relationship problems that need to be addressed. "Getting help from an outside professional can certainly help to balance out the equation and assist with negotiations of this type, and/or other underlying issues that prevent partners from connecting and communicating," Ghose says.

When it comes to kink, the bottom line is being willing to communicate with an open mind and heart. It's about coming to sex with a sense of curiosity and a willingness to take chances. We won't always have the same likes and dislikes as our partners, but having room to figure out different things that get you going can be a grand adventure.

## HOW TO GET STARTED WITH KINK SCENES THAT INVOLVE A PARTNER

Assuming your partner wasn't a "fuck no" on talking about kink and is interested in giving some of this play a try, it's time to co-create scenes and execute them together. What could be more wholesome?

Follow these four simple and easy steps.

### Step 1: Having conversations about where you land on the Dom/sub scale

Do the BDSM test together to figure out where you both land on the Dom/sub scale. In my clinical experience, there has rarely been a person who hasn't been at least a little bit kinky. No, that's a lie, actually. I've never had a client who couldn't find something on there that they would be willing to try. Having a better understanding of where you both fall on the kink spectrum can be an eye-opening experience that leads to deeper conversations about desire.

### Step 2: Talk about your specific fantasies

Get real about fantasies—both of your fantasies. Like I mentioned above, conversations surrounding our desires should be a two-way street. Everyone's feelings and interests must be respected for this to work. It doesn't mean you have to act on everything, but being open to discussion is critical if you ever want the opportunity to explore anything in real life. We all just want to feel seen and understood.

Get specific. For instance, if you're interested in spanking, are you the one who wants to be spanked, or do you want to do the spanking? How does your partner feel about spanking, and what role do they see themselves playing in said spanking scene?

BDSM and kink aren't hot unless everyone is enjoying it—at least to some extent. It might not be your partner's thing to spank you, but it is important that they enjoy it because you enjoy it. And I do mean "enjoy" with an emphasis on *joy*. There has to be joy in the play—otherwise, it, for lack of a better word, sucks. It's not about the dominant partner doing whatever they want to the submissive partner, willy-nilly. It's about both partners getting what they want out of the scene.

Try doing the Fantasy vs. "in real life" exercise together. It can be such a great way to get started on what you want a scene to look like. Time to get vulnerable, baby!

### Step 3: Starting your play slowly and intentionally

Always, always, always take things slowly when you're playing. Have your safe word at the ready and be prepared to say it/hear it at any time.

Don't tie your partner's arms and legs to the bed, throw on a blindfold, and pop in a ball gag on the first go with bondage. This could result in a massive panic attack. You want to begin with simple things and work yourselves to more advanced activities, should you want to.

For BDSM, I suggest starting by using flat palms to give or receive spankings on the bottom. Next, try tying your or your partner's wrists together during sex. Be sure to review Chapter 6: Physical Safety together before trying this.

You do not need to buy a lot of crazy stuff to try BDSM or kink. If you break the bank on a bespoke leather corset and then decide you're not that into bondage after all, what do you do then? You can't exactly donate it to a charity shop. Some kinks and fetishes don't even require gear—it's dependent on what you're both open to trying.

You can use all kinds of things around the house as makeshift BDSM gear. A wooden kitchen spoon is excellent for spanking. Use a cotton T-shirt as a blindfold and a necktie or pair of stockings to make handcuffs. Ice cubes work for temperature play. You can have a lot of fun with the things you already have.

### Step 4: Review the experience with your partner and plan for next time

Don't forget the aftercare! See how you feel about it and discuss your feelings after the fact. I suggest taking some time to cuddle and relax before chatting. Just be sure you don't go to bed without connecting. It's important to check in and assess your emotions before, during, and after BDSM of any kind.

If you want to do a scene again, talk about it. Figure out what worked for you, what didn't work for you, and maybe even what turned you off. If you didn't like the play at all, be open about this. It's OK to not want to try it again, and it's OK to want to try the play in a different way. Stay open-minded, but never do something just to please a partner. All sex should be fun, even when it stings a little (*wink wink*).

And it is as straightforward as that, my kink curious folx. Bringing a partner into play isn't all that complex; it just takes some empathy and patience. You've got this. I believe in you.

**AGONY AUNT QUESTION AND ANSWER: Can a lack of kinky compatibility end a relationship?**

**Q** *Dear Gigi,*

*I have an interest in alien implantation, and my partner doesn't. I'm not sure if it's a fetish, but it might be. It's definitely a strong desire. She doesn't even want to try it out with me. She thinks it's too weird. Does a lack of kinky compatibility mean my relationship won't work?*

*Alien Girl*

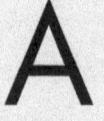

**A** Dear Alien Girl,

Whether or not a kink will end a relationship entirely depends on the couple's willingness to explore, in addition to how important kink is to the person who enjoys it. If your alien implantation fetish is something you absolutely need in your relationship to be sexually satisfied, you have to communicate that with your partner.

Normally, I would suggest finding a compromise here if your partner were open to exploring this. I'd say you could try playing out this fantasy sometimes, but not all the time. Maybe you could use an ovipositor dildo once in a while—you know, that kind of creative exploration.

But since your partner isn't open to doing that, I would suggest another option here. A secret option 2, if you will. Perhaps you can negotiate ways in which you can explore your kink without them. This could be in a non-monogamous way or with a professional kink expert whom you visit.

There are plenty of ways to make this work, but it won't be doable for everyone. It takes a willingness to be courageous and to try to find ways that work for everyone involved. If it turns out the kink is more important than the relationship and you can't find common ground, it may be time to rethink this particular relationship. This isn't a bad thing, but for many kinky people, it is central to who they are as a sexual human being—and when a partner doesn't understand that, it can be very challenging (for both people).

If your partner is unwilling to engage in this particular fetish, but they are into others you have, would that be something you could live with? Or perhaps there is some common fantasy you both share that could bridge this gap?

A lot of vanilla-leaning people can find they have kinks

they didn't know about. In such a sex-repressed culture, we aren't taught to explore the shadow side of our desires. This is worth exploring.

If the relationship is very important to you and you want to explore this further, seek an outside person. I'd see a kink-affirming professional—a coach or a therapist who works with kink as a specialty (like me!) to have an outside party help you find common ground and negotiate boundaries.

Is this relationship ending? Only you can answer that question. Figure out what is possible and what isn't, and then ask yourself: Can I live a full, rich, beautiful erotic existence within those boundaries? You'll know when you get there.

I hope this helps you find your way. Your fetish sounds awesome, by the way. How fun and creative that must be! I truly love it for you and hope you get to explore it.

XOXO Auntie Gigi

## Chapter 14 recap

Chapter 14 got right to the point: How can we start having these conversations with a partner—and how can we start to play together in a way that feels safe and authentic?

It turns out that taking a partner on a kink journey is all about bringing together the knowledge you've gained throughout the rest of the book. We focused mostly on opening conversations with more vanilla-leaning partners because those can be the trickiest kinds of relationships to navigate when we have a kink.

The takeaways: Get consent for the conversation, invite an open, two-way dialogue about fantasy, and go slowly when you start to play.

Last, we looked into a reader question about alien implantation fetish (so fun!), and thought critically about an uncomfortable yet necessary query: Can a fetish end a relationship? The answer: There are ways to work with a fetish that feels good for both partners, but it can also be a breaking point for some couples. And that's a valid reason to end a partnership.

## JOURNAL PROMPTS AND CONVERSATION STARTERS

These prompts are designed to get your conversation started. You're welcome to talk openly with each other or take some time to reflect (either in your head, in writing, or in a format that works for you) and then come back to the discussion. Reflect together on the questions once you've had a bit of time to process them. I recommend 10–15 minutes.

1. Ask your partner: Tell me about a fantasy you have.

2. What is your peak turn-on when it comes to sex?

3. Do you see yourself as more of a Dom or a sub? Why?

4. As we've opened the conversation around kink, what intrigues you? What scares you? What excites you?

5. If we were to explore some more adventurous sex, what might that look like for you in an ideal world?

# EXERCISES

## EXERCISE 1: Yes, No, Maybe lists—partner edition

You're very familiar with the Yes, No, Maybe list—and now it's time to add your partner. Grab the lists and take 10–15 minutes to do them separately. Then, come back together and see where there might be an overlap. Take some time to pick out kinks that are particularly intriguing and discuss what that might look like for the two of you. Try to choose two or three that are your most exciting and give them a try!

## EXERCISE 2: Creating a kinky sex menu

You're free to write your menu out or even draw it. It's all about what works for you and your partner. Making a menu can give you a solid way to communicate what you want from a scene at any given time.

**Step 1:** Think about past sexual experiences that you've had (we did this already in the "themes of kink" exercise in Chapter 10). Pick out a few of the things you enjoyed. Check for overlap with your partner. Put them into a column. These will serve as a first course.

**Step 2:** Revisit your Yes, No, Maybe lists and grab all the overlapping "Yeses." These will serve as a second course.

**Step 3:** Revisit your Yes, No, Maybe lists and grab any overlapping "Maybes." These will serve as a dessert.

**Step 4:** Before designing a scene, take a look at your menu. What would you like to be served during this experience? Discuss and choose accordingly.

**Step 5:** Have fun! You can come back to your menu—and even update it—anytime you want.

## KINK CURIOUS: FINAL THOUGHTS

What more can I even say? I've shared all I know about kink with you. What an absolute dream it has been to be on this journey alongside your brave self. Throughout my decade of experience in the sexual wellness world, kink will forever be the center of my fascination. It's been such a pleasure to be able to share with you the wisdom I've gained through so many years of study and practice.

I hope throughout these pages that you've gleaned some helpful advice and practical tips—but most of all, I hope you feel more centered and grounded in your kinkiness. I hope you feel more like yourself and freer in your desires.

Kink is a beautiful and artful way of looking at the vast and bountiful landscape of human sexuality. Exploring it can open our minds and bodies to the vast human capacity for pleasure. We all deserve that.

Don't forget about our journey together. Let this book be a continuous resource. You're always welcome here in these pages. If you're ever feeling unsteady, confused, unsure, or a tingling of shame, the exercises and journal prompts from this book can help you find your way. There may even come a time when you feel like your entire kinky personality might be shifting into something new. No matter how kinky we are, no matter how resolute in our desires, we're always going to be kink curious.

Thank you for being here with me. I'm so grateful for you and the time you've given to read this book and learn about yourself. I love you very much.

XOXO Auntie Gigi

# FURTHER READING AND RESOURCES

## KINKY BOOKS

*Playing Well With Others: Your Field Guide to Discovering, Navigating and Exploring the Kink, Leather and BDSM Communities*, by Mollena Williams-Haas and Lee Harrington

*50 Shades of Kink*, by Tristan Taormino

*Authentic Kink: Create Your Best Experience* (Workbook), by Princess Kali

*Superfreaks: Kink, Pleasure, and the Pursuit of Happiness*, by Arielle Greenberg

*The Ultimate Guide to Kink: BDSM, Role Play and the Erotic Edge*, by Tristan Taormino

*Why Are People Into That?*, by Tina Horn

*Tell Me What You Want*, by Justin Lehmiller

*When Someone You Love Is Kinky*, by Dossie Easton

## KINKY WEBSITES

Beducated

Climax

Erika Lust

OMGYes

Kink Academy

## KINKY PODCASTS

Come As You Are

Come Curious

Doin' It

In Touch

LoveBites

Private Parts Unknown

Sex Out Loud

Savage Lovecast

Sex and Psychology

Sexology Podcast

Why Are People Into That?

## KINKY PRACTITIONERS AND WORKSHOPS

Julieta Chiara: www.julietachiara.com/store

Eva Oh: www.eva-oh.com

Venus Cuffs: www.venuscuffs.com

Dirty Lola: https://dirtylola.com

Mistress Malissia and Mistress Mindset: www.mistressmindset.com

## KINKY SEX PARTIES

JoyRide: www.joyriderave.com

Torture Garden: www.instagram.com/torturegardenclub

Club Verboten: https://klubverboten.com

## RESOURCES FOR TRANS AND NON-BINARY LEARNING

*Disclosure* on Netflix: www.netflix.com/title/81284247

*Fucking Trans Women*: http://fuckingtranswomen.org

*Gender: A Graphic Guide*, by Meg-John Barker

*Gender Euphoria*, by Laura Kate Dale

*Girl Sex 101*, by Allison Moon

*Nerve Endings: The New Trans Erotic*, by Tobi Hill-Meyer

*Queer Sex*, by Juno Roche

Blueheart Sex and Relationship Therapy app and website: www.blue
heart.io

Adventuring with Pride (Queer Dnd supplement): https://adventuring
withpride.com

*Trans Sex: A Guide for Adults*, by Kelvin Sparks

*Take Me There: Trans and Genderqueer Erotica*, edited by Tristan Taormino

Trans Safer Sex Guide: http://hrc-assets.s3-website-us-east-1.amazonaws.
com//files/assets/resources/Trans_Safer_Sex_Guide_FINAL.pdf

...F@#king Trans Women blog, by Natalie Reed: http://freethought
blogs.com/nataliereed/2012/05/30/fking-trans-women

Sexplanations with Dr. Lindsey Doe: www.youtube.com/user/
sexplanations

*Not Your Mother's Meatloaf: A Sex Education Comic Book*, by Saiya Miller
and Liza Bley

## RESOURCES FOR UNLEARNING SHAME AND PURITY CULTURE

*Pure: Inside the Evangelical Movement That Shamed a Generation of Young Women and How I Broke Free,* by Linda K. Klein

*Sluts: The Truth About Slut Shaming,* by Beth Ashley

*Deconstructing My Religion* documentary: www.youtube.com/watch?v=gy9IilwCgBY

# BIBLIOGRAPHY

## INTRODUCTION

James, E.L. (2024) *Kinky History: A Rollicking Journey Through Our Sexual Past, Present, and Future*. New York: TarcherPerigee, Penguin Random House.

## CHAPTER 1

Richters, J., de Visser, R.O., Rissel, C.E., Grulich, A.E., and Smith A.M.A. (2008) 'Demographic and psychosocial features of participants in bondage and discipline, "sadomasochism" or dominance and submission (BDSM): Data from a national survey.' *The Journal of Sexual Medicine*, 5(7), 1660–1668. https://doi.org/10.1111/j.1743-6109.2008.00795.x

## CHAPTER 3

Joyal, C.C., Cossette, A., and Lapierre, V. (2014) 'What exactly is an unusual sexual fantasy?' *The Journal of Sexual Medicine*. Available at: https://onlinelibrary.wiley.com/doi/abs/10.1111/jsm.12734

Lehmiller, J. (2022) *Tell Me What You Want: The Science of Sexual Desire and How It Can Help You Improve Your Sex Life*. London: Robinson.

Strong, R. (2024) *Most Common Male Sex Fantasies (and How to Share Them With Your Partner)*. AskMen. Available at: www.askmen.com/sex/sex_fantasies/common-sex-fantasies.html

## CHAPTER 4

Cromie, W.J. (2002) 'Pleasure, pain activate the same part of the brain.' *Harvard Gazette*. Available at: https://news.harvard.edu/gazette/story/2002/01/pleasure-pain-activate-same-part-of-brain

Eveleth, R. (2014) 'Americans are more into BDSM than the rest of the world.' *Smithsonian Magazine*. Available at: www.smithsonian mag.com/smart-news/americans-are-more-bdsm-rest-world-180949703

Lehmiller, J. (2022) *Tell Me What You Want: The Science of Sexual Desire and How It Can Help You Improve Your Sex Life*. Robinson.

Martin, W. (2019) *Untrue: Why Nearly Everything We Believe About Women, Lust, and Infidelity Is Wrong and How the New Science Can Set Us Free*. New York: Little, Brown Spark.

Sagarin, B., Cutler, B., Cutler, N., Lawler-Sagarin, K.A., and Matuszewich, L. (2009) 'Hormonal changes and couple bonding in consensual sadomasochistic activity.' *Archives of Sexual Behavior*, 38(2), 186–200. Available at: https://doi.org/10.1007/s10508-008-9374-5

Trafton, A. (2017) *Scientists Identify Brain Circuit that Drives Pleasure-inducing Behavior*. MIT News Available at: https://news.mit.edu/2017/brain-circuit-pleasure-inducing-behavior-0322

**CHAPTER 5**

Cornier, J.R. (2019) *Hanky Panky: An Abridged History of the Hanky Code*. The History Project. Available at: https://historyproject.org/news/2019-04/hanky-panky-abridged-history-hanky-code-0

GLBT Historical Society (n.d.) *Primary Source Set: Leather*. GLBT Historical Society. Available at: www.glbthistory.org/primary-source-set-leather

Sprott, R.A. (2023) 'The intersection of LGBTQ+ and kink sexualities: a review of the literature with a focus on empowering/positive aspects of kink involvement for LGBTQ+ individuals.' *Current Sexual Health Reports*, 15(2), 107–112. https://doi.org/10.1007/s11930-023-00360-3

**CHAPTER 6**

American Sexual Health Association (2025) *STDs A–Z*. The American Sexual Health Association. www.ashasexualhealth.org/stds_a_to_z

CDC (n.d.) *Self Testing for HIV*. CDC. Available at: www.cdc.gov/hiv/testing/self-testing.html

CDC (2016) *Chlamydia Treatment and Recovery*. Centers for Disease
Control and Prevention. Available at: www.cdc.gov/chlamydia/
about/#cdc_disease_basics_treatment-treatment-and-recovery

CDC (2017) *Genital Herpes—CDC Fact Sheet*. Centers for Disease Control
and Prevention. Available at: www.cdc.gov/herpes/about/?CDC_
AAref_Val=https://www.cdc.gov/std/herpes/stdfact-herpes.htm

CDC (2019) *New CDC Report: STDs Continue to Rise in the U.S.* Centers for
Disease Control and Prevention. Available at: www.cdc.gov/nchhstp/
newsroom/2019/2018-STD-surveillance-report-press-release.html

CDC (2023) *Sexually Transmitted Infections*. Centers for Disease Control
and Prevention. Available at: www.cdc.gov/sti

Pinkerton, S.D. and Abramson, P.R. (1997) 'Effectiveness of condoms
in preventing HIV transmission.' *Social Science & Medicine*, 44(9),
1303–1312. Available at: www.sciencedirect.com/science/article/abs/
pii/S0277953696002584

Sagarin, B.J., Cutler, B., Cutler, N., Lawler-Sagarin, K.A. *et al.* (2008)
'Hormonal changes and couple bonding in consensual
sadomasochistic activity.' *Archives of Sexual Behavior*, 38(2), 186–200.
Available at: https://doi.org/10.1007/s10508-008-9374-5

WebMD (2024) *Rehab after Heart Attack May Help Recovery*. WebMD
& School of Public Health at Tel Aviv University. Available
at: www.webmd.com/sex-relationships/news/20200923/
had-a-heart-attack-resuming-sex-soon-after-might-be-healthy#1

## CHAPTER 7

Crown Prosecution Service (2023) *What Is Consent?* Crown Prosecution
Service. Available at: www.cps.gov.uk/sites/default/files/documents/
publications/what_is_consent_v2.pdf

Herbenick, D., Fu, T.-C., Wright, P., Paul, B., Gradus, R., *et al.* (2020)
'Diverse sexual behaviors and pornography use: Findings from a
nationally representative probability survey of Americans aged 18
to 60 Years.' *Journal of Sexual Medicine*, 17(4), 623–633. Available at:
https://pubmed.ncbi.nlm.nih.gov/32081698

Herbenick, D., Fu, T.-C., Eastman-Mueller, H., Thomas, S., Svetina Valdivia, D., *et al.* (2022). 'Frequency, Method, Intensity, and Health Sequelae of Sexual Choking Among U.S. Undergraduate and Graduate Students.' *Archives of Sexual Behavior*, 51(6), 3121–3139. doi:https://doi.org/10.1007/s10508-022-02347-y.

Hou, J., Huibregtse, M.E., Alexander, I.L., Klemsz, L.M., Fu, T.-C., *et al.* (2023). 'Association of Frequent Sexual Choking/Strangulation with Neurophysiological Responses: A Pilot Resting-State fMRI Study.' *Journal of Neurotrauma*. doi:https://doi.org/10.1089/neu.2022.0146.

Lawson, K. (2018) 'Half the country doesn't have a legal definition of consent.' *Vice*. Available at: www.vice.com/en/article/bj3p35/state-definition-of-consent-legislation

Nagoski, E. (2023) 'Consent and "Enthusiastic Maybe."' Come As You Are Podcast. Pushkin. Available at: www.pushkin.fm/podcasts/come-as-you-are/consent-and-enthusiastic-maybe

Planned Parenthood (2025) *Sexual Consent*. Planned Parenthood. Available at: www.plannedparenthood.org/learn/relationships/sexual-consent

## CHAPTER 8

McGreal, S.A. (2013) 'BDSM, personality, and mental health.' *Psychology Today*. Available at: www.psychologytoday.com/gb/blog/unique-everybody-else/201307/bdsm-personality-and-mental-health

Ten Brink, S., Coppens, V. Huys, W., and Morrens, M. (2020) 'The psychology of kink: A survey study into the relationships of trauma and attachment style with BDSM Interests.' *Sexuality Research and Social Policy*, 18, 1–12. Available at: https://link.springer.com/article/10.1007/s10508-024-02829-1

van der Kolk, B. (2015) *The Body Keeps the Score*. Penguin Random House

## CHAPTER 9

Jori (2019) *The Four Corners of Eroticism*. Flow House Therapy. Available at: https://www.joriadler.com/hidden/2020/2/10/the-four-corners-of-eroticism

Morin, J. (1995) *The Erotic Mind*. Headline.

Neves, S. (2021) *Compulsive Sexual Behaviours: A Psycho-Sexual Treatment Guide for Clinicians*. Routledge.

## CHAPTER 11

Lehmiller, J. (2020). *TELL ME WHAT YOU WANT: the science of sexual desire and how it can help you improve your sex life*. S.L.: Da Capo Press.

## CHAPTER 10

Moskowitz, D.A. and Roloff, M.E. (2017) 'Recognition and construction of top, bottom, and versatile orientations in gay/bisexual men.' *Archives of Sexual Behavior*, 46(1) 273–285. https://link.springer.com/article/10.1007/s10508-016-0810-7

## CHAPTER 13

Maczkowiack, J. and Schweitzer, R.D. (2019) Postcoital dysphoria: Prevalence and correlates among males. *Journal of Sex & Marital Therapy*, 45(2) 128–140. https://doi.org/10.1080/0092623X.2018.1488326